TOWARDS COMMUNITY
MENTAL HEALTH

TAVISTOCK

The International Behavioural and Social Sciences Library

HEALTH & SOCIETY
In 12 Volumes

TOWARDS COMMUNITY
MENTAL HEALTH

EDITED BY JOHN D SUTHERLAND

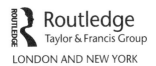

LONDON AND NEW YORK

First published in 1971 by
Tavistock Publications Limited

Published in 2001 by
Routledge
2 Park Square, Milton Park, Abingdon, Oxfordshire OX14 4RN
711 Third Avenue, New York, NY 10017

First issued in paperback 2014

Routledge is an imprint of the Taylor and Francis Group, an informa business

The publishers have made every effort to contact authors/copyright holders
of the works reprinted in the *International Behavioural and Social Sciences
Library*. This has not been possible in every case, however, and we would
welcome correspondence from those individuals/companies we have been
unable to trace.

These reprints are taken from original copies of each book. In many cases
the condition of these originals is not perfect. The publisher has gone to
great lengths to ensure the quality of these reprints, but wishes to point
out that certain characteristics of the original copies will, of necessity, be
apparent in reprints thereof.

British Library Cataloguing in Publication Data
A CIP catalogue record for this book
is available from the British Library

Towards Community Mental Health
ISBN 0-415-26433-2
Health & Society: 12 Volumes
ISBN 0-415-26509-6
The International Behavioural and Social Sciences Library
112 Volumes
ISBN 0-415-25670-4

ISBN 13: 978-1-138-86743-7 (pbk)
ISBN 13: 978-0-415-26433-4 (hbk)

Contributors

Elizabeth BOTT, M.A., PH.D.
Psychoanalyst and social anthropologist

Barbara BUTLER, M.A.
Lecturer in Applied Social Studies,
Bedford College, University of London

Geoffrey GORER, M.A., F.R.A.I.
Social anthropologist

Elliott JAQUES, M.A., M.D., PH.D.
Professor and Head of Department of Social Institutions,
Brunel College, University of London

Ben MORRIS, B.SC., ED.B.
Professor, Institute of Education, University of Bristol

Herbert PHILLIPSON, M.A., F.B.PS.S.
Chief Psychologist, Tavistock Clinic, London

John D. SUTHERLAND, C.B.E., PH.D., D.P.M., F.R.C.P.E.
Consultant in Psychotherapy, Department of Psychiatry,
University of Edinburgh; formerly Medical Director,
Tavistock Clinic, London

D. W. WINNICOTT, F.R.C.P. (Lond.)
Formerly President of the British Psycho-Analytical Society

Towards Community Mental Health

Edited by
JOHN D. SUTHERLAND

TAVISTOCK PUBLICATIONS
London · New York · Sydney · Toronto · Wellington

First published in 1971
by Tavistock Publications Limited
2 Park Square, Milton Park, Abingdon, Oxon, OX14 4RN
Editorial matter © John D. Sutherland
in 11 pt Garamond 1 pt leaded
by Butler and Tanner Ltd,
Frome and London

ISBN 0 422 73380 6

Distributed in the USA
by Barnes & Noble, Inc.

Contents

Introduction

JOHN D. SUTHERLAND

That 'mental health' was emerging as a new goal comparable with some of the master-values that have inspired various eras in our history, was suggested by Dicks (1950) twenty years ago. Since then, the subject has become part of our scene with a proliferation of associations and programmes devoted to improving mental health and, above all, with television bringing home to the public the great range of the psychiatric disorders and of the endeavours to treat and prevent them. This greater familiarity, however, is far from the acceptance of mental health as a master-value. On the contrary, there is a persistent and widespread tendency to restrict its import to those matters traditionally the concern of psychiatrists and the caring professions. It is for this reason that many have wished for another term. Yet, in spite of innumerable attempts to find an alternative, 'mental health' has remained, perhaps reflecting an unconscious appreciation that these are the right words in spite of the common narrowing of their meaning – that they do signify a master-value.

The aspirations within the larger concept are plain. Can man, with the knowledge he has gained of how he grows and is maintained as a person in his society, put this knowledge to use so that he may realize more of his potential? Early gains in the first decades of our century raised many false hopes – ludicrous oversimplifications, from the retrospective standpoint of today. Understanding has progressed steadily and perhaps our most valuable advances are in a greater realism about the complexity of man's personal nature. Our increased knowledge is also shedding light on some of the thorniest of the problems in this task, viz, the resistances to the acceptance of man's nature – what Bion (1962) has referred to so arrestingly and yet with such depressing accuracy as our 'hatred' of learning about ourselves. In this conflict, we have seen, oddly enough, science and religion with all the institutionalization of their stereotypes, as Dicks puts it, united Canute-like against the tide of the facts. But the voice of reason eventually gets its hearing. One of our sharpest theologians, Dr Ian Ramsey, the Bishop of Durham, in a recent lecture (1970) remarked on 'the devastating contrast between an ineffective, harsh theology, a polished cistern which contains no water, no living water, and the knowledge and skills of the Behavioural Sciences which seem to minister so obviously and creatively to the spirit of man'. Almost at the same time, and from the key position in British psychiatry, Sir Denis Hill (1970) has challenged psychiatrists and psychologists on their restrictive views of science and their exclusive concentration on mechanisms underlying behaviour while ignoring the whole phenomena of meaning and its manifestly central role in man's personal behaviour.

If the urgency of our need to know more of ourselves as persons has been denied by our individual and institutional resistances, the technological revolution going on apace is breaking through these barriers in disturbing ways. The current changes in our society are great enough to warrant the sociologists' description of them as a movement into a new 'post-industrial society'. In a penetrating analysis of its implications for the individual, Trist (1968) remarks that the steps we take with regard to the welfare and development of people during the next few decades will be critical. What is most characteristic of the society into which we are now moving is the entirely new degree of interdependence of individuals and organizations. This vastly increased interrelatedness is leading to situations that inevitably challenge existing beliefs and values within the core of the individual and in the institutions that shape him and are in turn shaped by him. For instance, organizational philosophies are shifting the emphasis from competitive relations and separate objectives to collaborative relations with linked objectives. Above all, this new interrelatedness leads to the perception of many social problems, such as poverty and crime, as major integrated problems requiring central planning rather than as an aggregate of separate elements to be tackled piecemeal. Central appraisals lead to 'ecological strategies' in which, for instance, crises are anticipated rather than responded to; measures are comprehensive with participation and confrontation of conflicts instead of being specific, requiring consent and covering up conflict. These new features forced upon us by the technological revolution demand that the individual move from such values as independence, achievement, and self-control to those of interdependence, self-actualization, and self-expression; from being one who endures a good deal of personal restriction, tension, and stress because of internal and external barriers, to becoming one who has a fuller and freer capacity for enjoyment.

In such a social scene, the relatively static notions of welfare as keeping people up to the standards needed by the industrial economy have to be complemented by the ideal of making personal development as rich as possible. The emphasis on the 'self' in these emergent values is noteworthy. The 'self' is the term we use for that core of the personality that preserves continuity in change and its integrity is what makes change acceptable. If this integrity of the self is threatened, change is resisted – often violently, as befits the defence of our most precious possession.

Several years after Dicks's paper, Marie Jahoda (1958) clarified some of the basic aspects implied by the term 'mental health'. She also brought out the different meanings it could have for different people and in different cultures. Nevertheless, we are on firmer ground than the considerations of cultural relativity might suggest. The new theoretical trends in psychoanalysis that had been initiated by Melanie Klein, and systematically developed by Fairbairn in his 'object relations theory of the personality', were helping to bridge the conceptual gap between what went on in the inner world of the individual and in the culture in which he and his family were embedded. It was the great merit of this approach that it conceived the structuring and functioning of the personality in terms of personal relationship systems. As with so many shifts in theoretical standpoints in the history of science, the new views could be seen as one expression of a fresh *Zeitgeist*. Other psychoanalysts, from their detailed studies of profound disturbances in the capacity for relationships, were independently reaching similar conclusions, e.g. Balint and Winnicott; and there was the exciting support this relationship-systems approach began to receive from the ethological theories of animal behaviour stimulated by the work of Lorenz. These concepts have been

notably applied to the psychoanalytic theory of child development by Bowlby. On the sociological side, the internalization
within the person of the relationships he experienced in the family
became a feature of the thinking of cultural anthropologists.
Cultural patterns were thus seen as interdependent with child-
rearing practices, and so cultural values and their influence on
the adult could be appraised on a more dynamic basis.

In the work of Parsons, Shils, and their colleagues, the structuring of the personality by the interactions within the family represented a most striking synthesis of the knowledge provided by
the psychoanalyst and that from the social scientist about the
forces from the social milien that impinge on the development
of the person.

The way in which these independent lines of thought confirmed
each other is remarkable – and a reassurance that appropriate
theoretical frameworks can be evolved for ordering this most
complex area of the individual as a person, with all that this
means, in his society. The essence of all this work is the emergence
of an adequate model of the development and functioning of the
person and of how culture mirrors and is mirrored by the inner
world of the individual.

The impetus towards synthesis, springing equally from those
psychoanalysts alive to social factors and from those social
scientists who accepted the full importance of psychodynamic
factors in the individual, has become a creative force in the theory
and practice of mental health programmes. Those who share in
this trend seek active relationships with sections of the community in which they may occupy a role closely analogous to
that of the analyst in his psychotherapeutic relationships. That
is to say, the efficacy of the part they play in any change process
arises from what they help to release, from the removal of inner
blockages to growth, and not from what they impose on the
thinking and actions of others. The criticism that such socially
active psychiatrists and allied colleagues take on omnipotent
powers is for the most part based on fantasies of the same kind that
attribute almost unlimited powers of suggestion to the analyst in
his psychotherapeutic work. (Most analysts have wished at times
that they did have such powers to influence behaviour in the relief
of suffering!) The fact is that change processes within community
institutions and ways are apt to evoke the same kind of anxiety

as arises in the individual who seeks to alter his established patterns of relating to himself and others.

The belief that the psychoanalyst and social scientist have an influential role in community mental health endeavours is not as yet widely shared amongst psychiatrists partly because few psychiatrists have the necessary training. For those who do, their contribution, though vital, is only one component in an 'ecological strategy'. The comprehensive nature of what must be tackled is well expressed by Trist:

' . . . at the higher level of complexity which characterizes the transition to post-industrialism a higher quality is required in all primary social units. By primary social units is meant the set of concrete social resources which exist in the life-space of the individual, i.e. the people and institutions with which he directly interacts and to which he contributes his own resources: his family, his work-place, the school his children attend, the particular community in which he resides, the services and amenities actually available to him: in sum, all those entities which compose his primary social world. The quality of those resources, in his case, determines for the individual his "quality of life", on which his welfare and development alike depend. The objective of taking the active role is to bring into being ecological systems able to maintain primary social worlds of high quality throughout a society. How to do this has now become the over-riding question as we move towards post-industrialism.'

Although written after the papers in the present volume were prepared, this statement aptly conveys the outlook of the Psychotherapy Section of the Royal Medico-Psychological Association in 1966 when its Executive Committee decided to devote the meetings of the 1966–67 Session to contributions on the theme 'Towards Community Mental Health'.

The speakers were not able to work together but were chosen because they shared broadly the basic principles of the kind of approach outlined. None of them would presume to have made a definitive statement. The papers represent the current working notions of a sample of people whose work seemed relevant, and as such had the limited aim of furthering an overall endeavour of daunting complexity. They appear now not in the order in which they were given, for that was governed by various practical considerations, but in a sequence that places them in a more logical progression of the contexts in which community mental health can be viewed.

As Chairman of the Section during their presentation, it was a great pleasure and a stimulating experience to listen to these papers, and I very much shared the wishes of the Committee of the Section that they should be made available to a wider audience. Because of the extraordinary pressures our psychiatrists are sub-jected to in providing services to relieve the more urgent suffering in our society, the image of psychiatry has become too much associated with the attempts to mitigate personal pain by drugs. Few psychiatrists are really satisfied with this role. Only when our society begins to grasp the real nature of its mental ill health, how-ever, will there be the opportunity to make adequate endeavours towards richer and healthier personal development for all. It is our hope that these papers will contribute, however modestly, to this objective.

REFERENCES

BION, W. R. (1962). *Learning from experience.* London: Heinemann.
DICKS, H. V. (1950). Towards our proper ethic. *Brit. J. med. Psychol.* **23**, 1.
HILL, Sir D. (1970). On mechanism and meaning. The Ernest Jones Lecture, March 1970.
JAHODA, M. (1958). *Current concepts of positive mental health.* New York: Basic Books.
RAMSEY, I. T. (1970). On not being judgmental. *Contact,* March.
TRIST, E. L. (1968). *The relation of welfare and development in the transition to post-industrialism.* Los Angeles: Sociotechnical Systems Division, Western Management Science Institute, University of California.

1　The Concept of a Healthy Individual

D. W. WINNICOTT

PRELIMINARIES

We use the words normal and healthy when we talk about people, and we probably know what we mean. From time to time we may profit from trying to state what we mean, at risk of saying what is obvious and at risk of finding we do not know the answer. In any case our standpoint moves on with the decades, so that a statement that suited us in the forties might seem to serve us badly in the sixties.

I shall not start off with quotations from those authors who have dealt with this same subject. Let me say at once that I have derived most of my concepts from those of Freud.

I hope that I shall not fall into the error of thinking that an individual can be assessed apart from his or her place in society. Individual maturity implies a movement towards independence, but there is no such thing as independence. It would be unhealthy for an individual to be so withdrawn as to feel independent and invulnerable. If such a person is alive, then there is dependence indeed! Dependence on mental nurse or family.

Nevertheless I shall study the concept of the health of the *individual*, because social health is dependent on individual health, society being but a massive reduplication of persons. Society cannot get further than the common denominator of individual health, and indeed cannot get so far, since society needs must carry its unhealthy members.

MATURITY AT AGE

In terms of development it can be said that health means maturity according to the maturity that belongs to the age of the individual. Premature ego development or premature self-awareness is no more healthy than is delayed awareness. The tendency towards maturation is part of that which is inherited. In a complex way (which has received much study) development, especially at the beginning, depends on a good-enough environmental provision. A good-enough environment can be said to be that which facilitates the various individual inherited tendencies so that development takes place according to inherited tendencies. Inheritance and the environment are each external factors if we speak in terms of the emotional development of the individual person, that is to say of psychomorphology. (I have wondered whether this term could be used instead of the clumsy use of the word psychology, prefixed by the word dynamic.)

It can usefully be postulated that the good-enough environment starts with a high degree of adaptation to individual infant needs. Usually the mother is able to provide this because of the special state she is in, which I have called primary maternal preoccupation. Other names have been given to this state but I am using my own descriptive term. Adaptation decreases according to the baby's growing need to experience reactions to frustration. In health the mother is able to delay her function of failing to adapt, till the baby has become able to react with anger rather than be traumatized by her failures. Trauma means the breaking of the continuity of the line of the individual's existence. It is only on a continuity of existing that the sense of self, of feeling real, and of being, can eventually be established as a feature of the individual personality.

INFANT–MOTHER INTERRELATIONSHIP

It is at the beginning, when the baby is living in a subjective world, that health cannot be described in terms of the individual alone. Later it becomes possible for us to think of a healthy child in an unhealthy environment, but these words make no sense at the beginning, till the baby has become able to make an objective assessment of actuality, and has become able to be clear about the not-me as distinct from the me, and between the shared *actual* and the phenomena of personal psychical reality, and has something of an internal environment.

I am referring to the two-way process in which the infant lives in a subjective world and the mother adapts in order to give each infant a basic ration of the *experience of omnipotence*. A living relationship is involved, essentially.

THE FACILITATING ENVIRONMENT

The facilitating environment and its progressive adjustments adaptive to individual needs could be isolated for study as a part of the study of health. Included would be the paternal functions supplementing the mother's functions, and the function of the family with its more and more (as the child becomes older) complex manner of introducing the reality principle while at the same time giving back the child to the child. Here, however, my aim is not to study the evolution of the environment.

EROTOGENIC ZONES

In the first half century of Freud any statement of health would need to be made in terms of the stage of id-establishment according to the successive predominance of erotogenic zones. This still has validity. The hierarchy is well known – starting with oral primacy, followed by anal and urethral primacies, and then followed by the phallic or 'swank' stage (the one that is so difficult for girl toddlers), and finally by the genital phase (three to five years) in which the *fantasy* includes all that belongs to adult sex. We are happy when a child fits in with this blueprint for growth.

Then in health the child reaches the characteristics of the latency period, in which there is no forward movement of id-positions and there is but sparse backing to id-impulse from the endocrine apparatus. The concept of health here is associated with the existence of a period of teachability, and in this period the sexes tend rather naturally to segregate themselves. These matters have to be mentioned because it is healthy to be six at six and ten at ten.

Then comes puberty, usually announced by a prepubertal phase in which a homosexual tendency may perhaps manifest itself. By the age of fourteen the boy or girl who has not stepped over into puberty may be inherently, and *in health*, thrown into a state of confusion and doubt. The word doldrums has been usefully applied here. Let me emphasize that it is not illness when a mid-puberty boy or girl flounders.

Puberty comes both as a relief and as an immensely disturbing phenomenon, one that we are only just beginning to be able to understand a little. At the present time boys and girls at puberty are able to experience adolescence as a period of growth in company with others in the same state; and the difficult task of sorting out what belongs to health and what belongs to illness in adolescence belongs to the post-war era in particular. The problems are, of course, not new.

One can only ask for those who are engaged in this task to put the emphasis on the solution of the theoretical problems rather than on the solution of the actual problems of the adolescents, who may, in spite of the inconvenience of their symptomatology, be best able to find their own salvation. The passage of time has significance here. The adolescent is not to be cured as if ill. I think this is an important part of the statement of health. This is not to deny that there can be illness during this age-period when adolescence is due.

Some adolescents suffer greatly, so that it is almost cruel to offer no help. At fourteen they are commonly suicidal, and theirs is the task of tolerating the interaction of several disparate phenomena – their own immaturity, their own puberty changes, their own idea of what life is about, and their own ideals and aspirations; add to this their personal disillusionment about the world of grown-ups – which for them seems to be essentially a world of compromise, of false values, and of infinite distraction from the main theme. As they leave this stage, adolescent boys and girls are beginning to feel real, to have a sense of *self* and of *being*. This is health. From being comes doing, but there can be no *do* before *be*, and this is their message to us.

We need not encourage adolescents who have personal difficulties, and who tend to be defiant while still dependent, and indeed they do not need encouragement. We remember that late adolescence is the age of exciting achievement in adventure, so that the emergence of a boy or girl from adolescence to the beginnings of an identification with parenthood and with responsible society is something that is good to watch. No one would claim that the word health is synonymous with the word ease. This is specially true in the area of conflict between society and its adolescent contingent.

If we proceed we begin to use a different language. This section started in terms of id-drives and ends up in terms of ego psychology. It is a great help to the individual when puberty can bring a potential for male potency and for the equivalent in girls, that is to say when full genitality is already a feature, having been reached in the reality of play at the age preceding the latency period. Nevertheless, boys and girls at puberty are not deceived into thinking that instinctual drives are all, and in fact they are essentially concerned with being, with being somewhere, with feeling real, and with achieving a degree of object constancy. They need to be able to ride the instincts rather than be torn to pieces by them.

Maturity or health in terms of the achievement of full genitality takes on a special form when the adolescent changes over into the adult who may become a parent. It is convenient when a boy who wishes to be like his father is able to dream heterosexually and to perform in full genital power; also when a girl, who wishes to be like mother, is able to dream heterosexually and experience genital orgasm in sexual intercourse. The test is: can sexual experience join up with liking and with the wider meanings of the word love?

Ill health in these respects is a nuisance, and inhibitions can be destructive and cruel in their operation. Impotence can hurt more than rape. Nevertheless, we do not feel contented nowadays with a statement of health in terms of id-positions. It is easier to describe the developmental process in terms of id-function than in terms of the ego and its complex evolution, yet the second method cannot be avoided. We must attempt to do this.

Where there is immaturity in the instinctual life then there is danger of ill health in the individual, in personality or character or behaviour; but one must be careful here to understand that sex can operate as a part-function so that, although sex may *seem* to be working well, potency and its female equivalent can be found to deplete, instead of enrich, the individual. But we are not easily taken in by these things, since we are not looking at the individual according to behaviour and surface phenomena. We are prepared to examine the personality structure and the relationship of the individual to society and to ideals.

Perhaps at one time psychoanalysts did tend *to think of health in terms of the absence of psychoneurotic disorder*, but this is no longer true. We now need more subtle criteria. We need not throw away what we used formerly when we now think in terms of freedom within the personality, of capacity for trust and faith, of matters of reliability and object constancy, of freedom from self-deception, and also of something that has to do with richness rather than poverty as a quality of personal psychical reality.

THE INDIVIDUAL AND SOCIETY

If we assume reasonable achievement in terms of instinct capacity then we see new tasks for the relatively healthy person. There is, for instance, his or her relationship to society – an extension of the family. Let us say that in health a man or woman is able *to reach towards an identification with society without too great a loss of individual or personal impulse*. There must, of course, be loss in the sense of control of personal impulse, but the extreme of identification with society with total loss of sense of self and self-importance is not normal at all.

If it is clear, then, that we are not contented with the idea of health as a simple absence of psychoneurotic disorder – that is, of disturbances relative to the progression of id-positions towards full genitality, and the organization of defence in respect of anxiety in interpersonal relationships – we can say in this context that health is not ease. The life of a healthy individual is characterized by fears, conflicting feelings, doubts, frustrations, as much as by the positive features. The main thing is that the man or woman feels he or she *is living his or her own life*, taking responsibility for action or inaction, and able to take credit for success and blame for failure. In one language it can be said that the individual has emerged from dependence to independence or to autonomy.

The thing that was unsatisfactory about the statement of health in terms of id-positions was the absence of ego psychology. A look at the ego takes us right back to the pregenital, preverbal stages of individual development, and to the environmental provision: adaptation geared to the primitive needs that are characteristic of earliest infancy.

At this point I tend to think in terms of HOLDING. This goes for the physical holding of the intra-uterine life, and gradually widens in scope to mean the whole of the adaptive care of the infant, including handling. In the end this concept can be extended to include the function of the family, and it leads on to the idea of the casework that is at the basis of social work. Holding can be done well by someone who has no intellectual knowledge of what is going on in the individual; what is needed is a capacity to identify, to know what the baby is feeling like.

In an environment that holds the baby well enough, the baby is able to make *personal development according to the inherited tendencies*. The result is a continuity of existence that becomes a sense of existing, a sense of self, and eventually results in autonomy.

DEVELOPMENT IN EARLY STAGES

Now I wish to look at what is going on in the early stages of personality development. Here the keyword is *integration*, which covers almost all the developmental tasks. Integration carries the baby through to unit status, to the personal pronoun I, to the number one; this makes possible I AM, which makes sense of I DO.

It will be appreciated that I am now looking in three directions at once. I am looking at infant care. Also I look at schizoid illness. In addition, I am seeking a way of stating what life can be about for healthy children and adults. In parenthesis, I would say that it is a characteristic of health that the adult does not stop developing emotionally.

I will take three examples. In the case of a baby, *integration* is a process, one that has its own pace and increasing complexity. In schizoid disorder, the phenomenon of *disintegration* is a feature, especially the fear of disintegration and the pathological organization of defences in the individual designed to give warning of disintegration. (Insanity is usually not a regression, which has an element of trust in it; it is rather a sophisticated arrangement of defences whose object is to prevent a repetition of disintegration.) Integration as a process of the kind that features in infant life reappears in the psychoanalysis of the borderline case.

In adult life, integration is enjoyed along with the ever-extending meaning of the term right up to and including integrity. Disintegration, in resting and in relaxation and in dreaming, can be allowed by the healthy person, and the pain associated with it accepted; especially because relaxation is associated with creativity, so that it is out of the *unintegrated* state that the creative impulse appears and reappears. Organized defence against disintegration robs the individual of the precondition for the creative impulse and therefore prevents creative living.[1]

[1] It is thought by some, as in Balint's paper (1952) discussing Khan, that much of the pleasure in the experience of art in one form or another arises from the

The Psychosomatic Partnership

A subsidiary task in infant development is that of psychosomatic indwelling (leaving the intellect out for the moment). Much of the physical part of infant care – holding, handling, bathing, feeding, and so on, is designed to facilitate the baby's achievement of a psyche–soma that lives and works in harmony with itself.

In psychiatry again, it is a feature of schizophrenia that there is only a loose connexion between the psyche (or whatever it may be called) and the body and its functions. The psyche may even be absent from the soma for a considerable period of time, or may be projected.

In health, the use of the body and all its functions is one of the enjoyable things, and this applies especially to children and to adolescents. So here again is a relationship between schizoid disorder and health. It is distressing that healthy persons may have to live in deformed or diseased or old bodies, or may be starving or in great pain.

Object-relating

Relating to objects can be looked at in the same way as psychosomatic coexistence and the wider issue of integration. Object-relating is something that the maturational process drives the baby to achieve, but cannot happen securely unless the world is presented to the baby well enough. The adapting mother presents the world in such a way that the baby starts with a ration of the

---

nearness to unintegration to which the artist's creation may safely lead the audience or viewer. So where the artist's achievement is potentially great, failure near the point of achievement may cause great pain to the audience by bringing them close to disintegration or the memory of disintegration, and leaving them there. The appreciation of art thus keeps people on a knife-edge, because achievement is so close to painful failure. This experience must be reckoned part of health.

[1] Here belongs another complication – the intellect, or the part of the mind that may become split off, and be exploited at great cost in terms of healthy living. A good intellect is no doubt a wonderful thing, so special to human beings, but there is no need for the intellect to be too closely linked in our minds with the idea of health. Study of the place of the intellect relative to the area I am discussing is an important subject, consideration of which would be out of place.

experience of omnipotence, this being the proper foundation for his or her later coming to terms with the reality principle. A paradox is involved here, in that in this initial phase the baby creates the object, but the object is already there, else he would not have created it. The paradox has to be accepted, not resolved.

Now let us carry this over to the fields of mental illness and to adult health. In schizoid illness, object-relating goes wrong; the patient relates to a subjective world or fails to relate to any object outside the self. Omnipotence is asserted by means of delusions. The patient is withdrawn, out of contact, bemused, isolated, unreal, deaf, inaccessible, invulnerable, and so on.

In health a great deal of life has to do with various kinds of object-relating, and with a 'to and fro' process between relating to external objects and relating to internal ones. In full fruition this is a matter of interpersonal relationships, but the residues of creative relating are not lost, and this makes every aspect of object-relating exciting.

Health here includes the idea of tingling life and the magic of intimacy. All these things go together and add up to a sense of feeling real and of being, and the experiences of feeding back into the personal psychical reality, enriching it, and giving it scope. The consequence is that the healthy person's inner world is related to the outer or actual world and yet is personal and capable of an aliveness of its own. Introjective and projective identifications are constantly taking place. It follows that loss and ill fortune (and illness, as I have said) may be more terrible for the healthy than for those who are psychologically immature or distorted. Health must be allowed to carry its own risks.

RECAPITULATION

At this stage of the argument we must burden ourselves with a consideration of our terms of reference. We need to decide whether to confine our consideration of the meaning of health to those who are healthy from the beginning, or to extend it to cover those who carry a germ of ill health and yet manage to 'make it' in the sense of reaching in the end a state of health that did not come easily and naturally. I feel we must include this latter category. I will very briefly describe what I mean.

Two Kinds of Person

I find it useful to divide the world of people into two classes. There are those who were never 'let down' as babies and who are to that extent candidates for the enjoyment of life and of living. There are also those who did suffer traumatic experience of the kind that results from environmental let-down, and who must carry with them all their lives the memories (or the material for memories) of the state they were in at moments of disaster. These are candidates for lives of storm and stress and perhaps illness.

We recognize the existence of those who lost grip of the tendency towards healthy development, and whose defences are organized in rigidity, the rigidity being itself a guarantee against forward movement. We cannot extend our meaning of the word health to cover this state of affairs.

There is a middle group, however. In a fuller exposition of the psychomorphology of health, we would include those who carry round with them experiences of unthinkable or archaic anxiety, and who are defended more or less successfully against remembering such anxiety, but who nevertheless use any opportunity that turns up to become ill and have a breakdown in order to approach that which was unthinkably terrible. The breakdown only seldom leads to a therapeutic result, but the positive element in the breakdown must be acknowledged. Sometimes the breakdown does lead to a kind of cure, and then the word health turns up again.

There seems to be a tendency towards healthy development that persists even here, and if these people in my second category can manage to hitch on to this tendency towards development, even if late, they may yet make good. We can then include these in among the healthy. Healthy by hook or by crook.

Flight to Sanity

We need now to remind ourselves that a flight to sanity is not health. Health is tolerant of ill health; in fact, health gains much from being in touch with ill health in all its aspects, especially the ill health called schizoid, and with dependence.

In between the two extremes of the first or lucky group and the second or unlucky group (in respect of early environmental provision) there is a big proportion of all persons who successfully hide a relative need for breakdown, but who do not actually break down unless existing environmental features trigger it off. These may take the form of a new version of the trauma, or it may be that a reliable human being has raised hopes.

So we ask ourselves the question: how wide a spectrum of these people who are making good in spite of what they carry round with them (genes, early let-downs, and unfortunate experiences) do we include among those who are healthy? We have to take into consideration the fact that in this group are many uncomfortable people whose anxiety propels them to exceptional achievement. They may be difficult to live with, but they push the world forward in some area of science, art, philosophy, religion, or politics. I do not have to decide the answer but I do have to be prepared for the legitimate question: what about the world's geniuses?

True and False

There is a special case of this awkward category, in which potential breakdown dominates the scene, that does not, perhaps, give us so much trouble. (But nothing in human affairs is clear cut, and who shall say where health stops and ill health takes over?) I refer to those people who have unconsciously needed to organize a false-self front to cope with the world, this false front being a defence designed to protect the true self. (The true self has been traumatized and it must never be found and wounded again.) Society is easily taken in by the false-self organization, and has to pay heavily for this. The false self, from our point of view here, though a successful defence, is not an aspect of health. It merges into the Kleinian concept of a manic defence – where there is a depression but this depression is denied, by unconscious process of course, so that the symptoms of depression appear as their opposites (up for down, light for heavy, white or luminous for dark, liveliness for deadness, excitement for indifference, and so on).

This is not health, but it has a healthy aspect in terms of holidays, and it also has a happy link with health, in that for ageing or old people the quickness and liveliness of the young is a perpetual, and surely legitimate, counter to depression. Seriousness has its link, in health, with the heavy responsibilities that come with age, responsibilities that the young wot not of, usually.

Here I need to mention the subject of *depression* itself – a price to pay for integration. It will not be possible for me to repeat here what I have written on the subject of the value of depression, or rather the health that is inherent in the capacity to be depressed, the depressed mood being near to the ability to feel responsible, to feel guilty, to feel grief, and to feel the full joy when things go well. It is true, however, that depression, however terrible, is to be respected as evidence of personal integration.

In ill health there are complicating destructive forces that when inside the individual favour suicide and when outside carry liability to delusions of persecution. I am not suggesting that these elements are part of health. Nevertheless, in a study of health it is necessary to include the seriousness akin to depression that belongs to individuals who have grown up in the sense of having become whole. It is in such persons that we can find richness and potential in a personality.

Omissions

I must omit the localized subject of the antisocial tendency. This is related to deprivation, that is to say, to a good era that came to an end at a phase in the child's growth when the child could know, but could not cope with, its results.

This is not the place to write about aggression. Let me say, however, that in the community it is the ill members who are compelled by unconscious motives to go to war and to attack as a defence against delusions of persecution, or else to destroy the world, a world that annihilated them, each one of them separately, in their infancy.

LIFE'S PURPOSE

I want finally to look at the life that the healthy person is able to live. What is life about? I do not need to know the answer, but we can agree that it is more nearly about BEING than about sex. Lorelei said: 'Kissing is all very well but a diamond bracelet lasts for ever' (Loos, 1935). Being and feeling real belong essentially to health, and it is only if we can take being for granted that we can get on to the more positive things. I contend that this is not just a value judgement, but that there is a link between individual emotional health and a sense of feeling real. No doubt the vast majority of people take feeling real for granted, but at what cost? To what extent are they denying a fact, namely that there could be a danger for them of feeling unreal, of feeling possessed, of feeling they are not themselves, of falling for ever, of having no orientation, of being detached from their bodies, of being annihilated, of being nothing, nowhere? Health is not associated with *denial* of anything.

The Three Lives

My last word must be about the three lives that healthy people live.

1. The life in the world, with interpersonal relationships as the key even to making use of the non-human environment.
2. The life of the personal (sometimes called inner) psychical reality. This is where one person is richer than another, and deeper, and more interesting when creative. It includes dreams (or what dream material springs out of).

With these two you are familiar, and it is well known that either may be exploited as a defence: the extrovert needs to find fantasy in living; and the introvert may become self-sufficient, invulnerable, isolated, and socially useless. But there is another area for human health to enjoy, one that is not easily referred to in terms of psychoanalytic theory.

3. The area of cultural experience.

Cultural experience starts as play, and leads on to the whole area of man's inheritance, including the arts, the myths of history, the slow march of philosophical thought and the mysteries of mathematics, and of group management and of religion.

Where do we place this third life of cultural experience? I think it cannot be placed in the inner or personal psychical reality because it is not a dream, it is a part of shared reality. But it cannot be said to be part of external relationships because it is dominated by dream. Also, of the three lives, it is the most variable; in some anxious restless people it has practically no representation, whereas in others this is the important part of human existence, where animals do not even start. For into this area come not only play and a sense of humour but also all the accumulated culture of the past five to ten thousand years. In this area the good intellect can operate. It is all a byproduct of health.

I have tried to work out where cultural experience is located, and I have tentatively made this formulation, that it starts *in the potential space between a child and the mother when experience has produced in the child a high degree of confidence in the mother*, that she will not fail to be there if suddenly needed.

Here I find I join up with Fred Plaut (1966), who used the word trust here as the key to the establishment of this area of healthy experience.

Culture and Separation

In this way health can be shown to have a relationship with living, with inner wealth, and in a different way with the capacity to have cultural experience.

In other words, in health there is no separation, because in the space–time area between the child and the mother, the child (and so the adult) lives creatively, making use of the materials that are available – a piece of wood or a late Beethoven quartet.

This is a development of the concept of transitional phenomena.

There is very much more that could be said about health, but I hope I have succeeded in giving the idea that I think a human being is unique. Ethology is not enough. Human beings have animal instincts and functions, and at times they look very much like animals. Perhaps lions are more noble, monkeys are more nimble, gazelles more graceful, snakes more sinuous, fishes more prolific, and birds more lucky because they are able to fly, but human beings are quite a thing on their own, and when they are healthy enough they do have cultural experiences superior to those of any animal (except perhaps whales and their relatives).

It is human beings who are likely to destroy the world. If so we can perhaps die in the last atomic explosion knowing that this is not health but fear; it is part of the failure of healthy people and healthy society to carry its ill members.

SUMMARY

What I hope I have done is to:

1. Use the concept of health as absence of psychoneurotic illness.

2. Link health with maturation ending with maturity.

3. Point out the importance of maturational processes that con-

cern the ego rather than those related to a consideration of id-positions in the hierarchy of erotogenic zones.

4. Link these ego processes with infant-care, schizoid illness, and adult health, using in passing the concepts of
    (a) integration
    (b) the psychosomatic partnership
    (c) object-relating
as examples of what obtains in the total scene.

5. Point out that we have to decide how far to include, and whether to include, those who reach to health in spite of handicaps.

6. Name the three areas in which human beings live, and suggest that it is a matter of health that some lives are valuable and effective, that some personalities are rich and creative, and that for some experience in the cultural area is the most important bonus that health brings.

7. Lastly, indicate not only that society depends for its health on the health of its members, but also that its patterns are those of its members reduplicated. In this way democracy (in one meaning of the word) is an indication of health because it arises naturally out of the family, which is in itself a construct for which healthy individuals are responsible.

REFERENCES

BALINT, M. (1952). Notes on the dissolution of object-representation in modern art. *Journal of Aesthetics and Art Criticism* **10** (4).
LOOS, ANITA (1935). *Gentlemen prefer blondes*. New York: Brentano.
PLAUT, F. (1966). Reflections about not being able to imagine.

2 Family and Crisis

ELIZABETH BOTT

In this paper I want to discuss how the immediate family is linked with society, and how these connexions affect its capacity to cope with certain stress situations.

By 'immediate' family I mean the social unit composed of mother, father, and children. It is also called 'nuclear' family, 'elementary' family, or sometimes just 'family' – all the terms are interchangeable.

It is now generally accepted by the 'helping' professions that one cannot understand an individual in isolation from his immediate family. At least this idea is accepted in theoretical terms, though it is not always acted on in practice. What is *not* understood or accepted so much is the place of the family itself in its social setting. In particular, comparatively little is known about the effects of the family's external social connexions on the family's internal relationships. It is this aspect of the family on which I want to concentrate. Most of my thesis is based on a study of ordinary families carried out at the Tavistock Institute some ten years ago (Bott, 1957), and on parts of a later study my husband and I carried out in the Kingdom of Tonga, a Polynesian island in the south Pacific. But when I come to discuss the family's responses to stress I shall have to go beyond my personal field experience.

One can learn something about the position of the immediate family in our own society by contrasting it with the position of the immediate family in other societies. In small-scale societies like Tonga, the immediate family is contained within a larger group composed partly of relatives and partly of friends and neighbours. Everybody knows everybody else. Because they all know each other and live together continuously, one does not encounter the sort of discontinuity we are so familiar with here, where a grandmother has one opinion, a neighbour another, a general practitioner has a third view, and a school doctor a fourth. In a small-scale society the equivalents of the grandmother, the neighbour, the general practitioner, and the school doctor would have ironed out their differences long ago – or if they could not manage that, they would at least know that disagreements existed.

When a family is contained in a larger group it gets a lot of emotional and material support. This is particularly noticeable at times of stress. When a Tongan father dies, for example, the psychic and social work of mourning must be carried out, but there are male relatives who can perform fatherly functions for the children, and the widow has close personal relationships with relatives who support her financially and emotionally. When children are orphaned, or when a family member becomes incapacitated through illness or old age, the effect on the family is not catastrophic. There is no need for orphanages, old peoples' homes, or mental hospitals. Households and families are large enough to carry one or two helpless people.

All this sounds idyllic but of course it is not. Support is accompanied by complete lack of privacy. Gossip is continual and usually vicious. The contrast between the situation in our society and a small-scale society was summed up for me by a young Tongan girl after she had lived in London for a year or so: 'I see now how you Europeans are different from us – no help, no gossip.' Or again: 'When you leave Tonga you feel free; when you reach England you feel lonely.'

I am not claiming that this sort of family system is better than ours, only that it is different; and further, that it is adapted to the economic and ecological conditions of life in a small-scale society just as our type of family structure is adapted to our more complex division of labour, to the necessity for physical mobility, and to the inevitable segregation of our social institutions.

In our society the immediate family is *not* contained within a larger group. But it is not isolated either. It is connected, through its individual members, with a lot of other groups and institutions. But these groups and institutions are not necessarily linked up with each other. The family thus lives in what I have called a *network*, not in a group, nor in a 'community' except in the loose geographical sense. The diagram represents the situation schematically.

This network formation has a considerable effect on the family's internal relationships. Compared with the situation in small-scale societies, families in our society have more privacy and more chance to work out their own *modus vivendi* without outside interference. Another difference is that when a family lives in a network, its members put all their emotional eggs in the family basket, so to speak. Outside there is discontinuity; inside there is

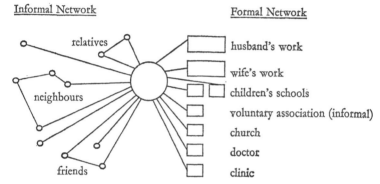

Informal Network   Formal Network

relatives

husband's work

wife's work

neighbours

children's schools

voluntary association (informal)

church

doctor

friends

clinic

continuity. Outside, you have various part identities – you are a colleague, a patient, a pupil, a friend: inside, you are you. In a small-scale society a man may be able to love his mother, respect his sister, hate his father's sister, and copulate with his wife. In our system he does all four with his wife – more rewarding perhaps, but also more difficult emotionally for both husband and wife. For the children, our family system is a pressure cooker. When there is a family row in a small-scale society, a child can wander off to visit an aunt for a few hours until things cool down at home. Our children have to stay with it, especially if it is winter time and the family lives in a small flat.

But not all families in our society have exactly the same sort of external network. Some networks are more connected than others, that is, more of the people the family know are independently related to one another. These differences apply particularly to the informal sector of the network, to relations among friends, neighbours, and relatives. Highly connected informal networks tend to be found in areas where, chiefly for economic reasons, many people in a neighbourhood have grown up and continued to live in the same place. Networks tend to become loose-knit where people move around a lot, which is the typical middle-class pattern (though many working class families move too, especially at the present time): one or two moves in childhood, one or two schools—often not in the same neighbourhood as one's home, then university, then two or three jobs each in a different place, then marriage and a flat, then a larger house or flat in another place. In each place one makes a few friends, but the friends in one context do not know the friends in the others. One loses touch with old friends and with nearly all one's relatives except for parents and possibly a sibling or two.

The main thing that emerged from our study of normal families at the Tavistock Institute was that the connectedness of the family's network was associated with the role-relationship between husband and wife. If the network is highly connected, husband and wife tend to have a segregated relationship – he lives his life, and she lives hers; there is a strict division of labour, and recreation tends to be separate. If their network is dispersed and loose-knit, husband and wife tend to have a joint relationship, that is, they are more likely to share tasks, activities, friends, recreation, and decisions; they believe that loyalty to one's spouse and one's immediate family should have priority over loyalty to anyone outside.

In the case of a family with a highly connected network, marriage is superimposed on a pre-existing set of relationships which are continued after the marriage. Both husband and wife can continue to get emotional support and sometimes material help from their previous networks – the wife chiefly from her relatives, the husband chiefly from friends. Their emotional investment in the marriage can afford to be less intense because it is not their only source of continuity and identity. Such families are a step nearer to the situation of the immediate family in a small-scale society.

Of course network connectedness is not the only factor in the role-relationship of husband and wife. The phase of marriage is also crucial: in the early days the relationship tends to be joint; after children are born it gradually becomes more segregated; and after children leave home it seems to remain comparatively segregated – though I am not at all sure of this point because we did not study this phase of marriage. The mode of relationship also varies radically according to the type of activity: important decisions tend to be joint, routine tasks segregated, and recreation the most variable activity of all and therefore in some ways the most useful in finding out what the family thinks their typical role-expectations are.

Changing from one type of network to another can assume the proportions of a crisis for a time. When a family with a connected network, say in Bermondsey or Bethnal Green, moves to a new housing estate, the wife, particularly, is up against it. She is cut off from her old network of mother and relatives and has not had much practice in developing friendships with strangers. There is no one to help her out, so she turns to her husband and, if they can both manage it, their relationship becomes more joint for a time. She may consult her general practitioner with vague physical disorders and general complaints of fatigue. If he probes into the situation he is likely to come to the conclusion that she is overdependent on her mother. This is quite right in a way, but it is not just a matter of individual personality. She is coping with a social situation with which the doctor, looking at her from the standpoint of his type of informal network, family ideology, and medical training, is quite unfamiliar.

But change in the other direction, from a dispersed to a close-knit network, can be equally painful. Some of my friends who were used to a dispersed network and a joint relationship moved to live permanently in Cambridge. The husbands soon got deeply involved with work and college politics, and at dinner parties used to retreat to one end of the room to talk shop, leaving the women to talk clothes, children, and the latest plays. 'Ghastly,' as one wife put it, 'just a lower middle-class suburb with intellectual whatnottery instead of privet hedges.'

Up to this point I have been dealing with my own research or personal experience. Now I want to discuss the way families react to certain crises, which means talking through my hat, or rather through other people's hats, since I have not done any research in the area concerned and most of the people who have studied these problems have not approached them from the point of view of the family in its network. In many cases they have dealt with the impact of a crisis on the members of the immediate family, and with the help provided by the formal helping agencies. But most research workers have not studied what use, if any, a crisis-ridden family makes of their informal network, their relatives, neighbours, and friends.

c

I am basing what I have to say partly on the work of Gerald Caplan (1961), but also on that of George Brown and his colleagues at the Social Psychiatry Research Unit of the Medical Research Council (see especially Brown *et al.*, 1966), on the work of Dennis Scott on the families of schizophrenics (Scott and Ashworth, 1965 and 1967), on Tilda Goldberg's studies (1967), on some of the work of Ronald Laing (Laing and Esterson, 1964), and on the work of Enid Mills (1962). And I am bearing in mind the work of John Sutherland (see chapter 5, this volume), Michael Balint (Balint and Balint, 1961), and others on the role of the specialist clinic in supporting and supervising other professional groups.

The word 'crisis' is confusing for a start. Caplan and his colleagues, the 'crisis theorists', define crisis as a temporary disorganization of an open system precipitated by a stress situation that overtaxes the system's capacity for internal adjustment and external adaptation. This is a very general definition, which can apply equally well to individuals or groups and can be used whenever equilibrium is disturbed, however grossly or slightly. There are the normal developmental crises of pregnancy, birth, the beastliness of toddlers, children starting school, adolescence, marriage, retirement, old age, and death. There are crises which happen to some people but not to others – catastrophic illness, sudden illness, accidents, deformities, unexpected bereavements, unemployment, unexpected separations, illegitimacy, divorce. The usefulness of Caplan's definition is that it provides a very general model within which different types of stress, crisis, and handling of crisis can be compared.

Unfortunately the word crisis has quite another connotation to many psychiatrists – it means the situation that arises when a psychiatric patient puts a brick through a window or threatens his mother with a knife. Such an event would fall within Caplan's definition, but the psychiatrist's usage would exclude many of Caplan's crises. I think we need a special term for the brick-throwing crisis – 'psychiatric crisis', perhaps, or 'explosive crisis'.

If one compares the family in our society with the family in a small-scale society, one finds a striking contrast in general ability to cope with crises, using the term in Caplan's sense. It is comparatively easy for a family in a small-scale society to cope with all the stress situations I have listed above because they can get so much help, both material and emotional, from relatives and friends. In fact, most of the events described above are not really defined as crises; they are the stuff of everyday life.

With us the situation is quite different. We tick over fairly nicely in ordinary circumstances, but the slightest change can upset our equilibrium completely. To take a very minor crisis with which I am sure everyone is familiar: I once found myself with all four members of my household incapacitated. My husband and my Tongan girl had influenza; both children had chicken-pox. As I struggled to open a tin of orange juice with one hand while the baby bit my shoulder and the other three invalids were calling for attention from their respective rooms, it suddenly struck me how different it would have been in Tonga. People would have just 'arrived' because they had heard about it. Meals would be prepared, I would be sent off for a rest, children would be comforted, and so on. Of course I would have been expected to provide food, tobacco, and presents, probably for a much longer period than the crisis lasted, but I would not have been alone.

Let us look briefly at the Tongan and English methods of coping with the birth of a baby, a normal developmental crisis. At the time of birth a young mother in Tonga is relieved of all responsibility for two to three months. Her only job is to lie down and make milk for the baby. Relatives cook meals, wash clothes, and walk around with the baby if he is irritable. The mother does not even have to organize it. Throughout she has continuity – the same people look after her during pregnancy, during childbirth, and afterwards. With the partial exception of the Maternity and Child Welfare Clinic, everyone gives her the same advice. In any case she has already looked after several babies and knows how to do it.

Contrast this with the position of the young mother in our society. Often she knows very little about babies. In pregnancy she starts with her general practitioner, then often moves on to hospital antenatal staff, to hospital delivery staff, to hospital maternity ward staff, and then back to her general practitioner and on to the Maternity and Child Welfare Clinic – none of these groups having any really close liaison with each other as far as the mother can see, and none being connected with her relatives, neighbours, and friends. On top of that someone has to get meals on time, clean, wash clothes, shop, cope with older children, feed the baby, and comfort him if he is fractious, especially at night. It seems to me small wonder that the symptoms of *post-partum* depression are more marked in our society. The somatic and emotional problems are probably much the same in any society – the sudden hormonal changes, the reawakening of conflicts with one's mother, the envy of the baby who receives all the care – but at least the mother in Tonga is not harassed by fatigue, household tasks, and the omnipresence of the clock.

What happens in our society to families when a child is born? Clinical workers often report that the wife turns to the husband to hold the situation, and sometimes say, quite rightly I think, that it is a bit hard to expect the husband to be husband, mother, cook/housekeeper, baby-walker, and amateur psychiatrist all at the same time. Many husbands are not cut out for it. But I think we really do not have enough systematic information on the use that different types of family make of their informal networks. How often are relatives called in and how helpful are they felt to be? What are the attitudes of the family to the mother and the mother-in-law as helpers, and are these purely individual reactions, or do they also depend on network formation and the role-relationship between husband and wife? Do people who get help from their relatives make less use, or more perfunctory use, of their general practitioner and the Maternity and Child Welfare Clinic? What sort of help, if any, is provided by neighbours and friends? Some answers to these questions have been provided by the research carried out by Jane Hubert of the Department of Anthropology at the London School of Economics and Political Science.

It seems to me that it would be useful to examine the various types of crisis situation from a threefold point of view: first, what happens inside the family; second, what use, if any, does the family make of their informal network; and third, what use do they make of the various formal institutions with which they are connected. The first and the third have been studied fairly intensively, especially by Caplan and his colleagues. The second, that is, the use families make of their informal networks, has not been examined so closely.

I want now to examine the effects of a drastic crisis: what happens when one of the family members becomes psychotic. I became interested in this problem when making a sociological study of a mental hospital, though I did not study the families directly, so that I have many questions to ask but few answers to provide.

First, what is the effect on the immediate family itself? The first point is that from the family's point of view psychosis is dreadful, a fact that one tends to forget if one deals with psychosis professionally all the time. In spite of the mental health propaganda of the press and of television programmes, psychosis still carries an enormous social stigma. If, in addition, the family confirm their fear that their patient has an illness that cannot be cured, that they are stuck with someone who is partly or wholly disabled and subject to recurrent hospitalizations, they face the prospect of living in a permanently abnormal state. As a family they are tainted, different from everyone else. Whatever explanation of the illness they adopt, the conclusions are disheartening. If the husband is ill, the wife may ask herself, consciously or unconsciously, what she has done to produce it or make it worse. If she adopts the hereditary hypothesis, she will worry about her children: 'Are they tainted?' The children ask themselves the same questions, 'Am I such a bad child that I have driven him mad? Is it going to happen to me? Will it happen to my children?' If a child is ill the parents may ask 'What have we done?' If they adopt the hereditary point of view they are carriers. 'Why him and not me?' they may ask, but also 'Thank God it is him and not me.' If the parents are old, they are sure to ask themselves 'What will happen to him when I die and there is no one who really cares about him?' Of course many of these ideas are too appalling to be openly discussed in the family or sometimes even thought about. The most primitive defences are likely to be brought into play to stop the family members suffering the full impact of the situation.

People who study the families of psychotics sometimes remark that the other family members are almost as crazy as the patient, and often assume that things have always been like this. But can we be so sure? Have the other members of the family driven the patient mad to save themselves, or are they displaying an eruption of psychotic defences against the full realization of the disaster that has overtaken them – or is it a bit of both? This question is not easily answered, especially as retrospective studies are notoriously unreliable. But the work of Searles (1958) and Dennis Scott

(Scott and Ashworth, 1965) in rediscovering positive family feeling through the transference in the treatment of schizophrenic patients and their families suggests that we could all afford to be more open-minded on the question.

Another finding about the response of the immediate family to psychotic illness has been their extraordinary devotion to the patient. They make many sacrifices on his behalf, sacrifices that sometimes go far beyond what is required by or for the patient. The bond is much stronger between parents and children than between husbands and wives. Spouses can cut their losses and get divorced; parents do not divorce their children so easily. And the work of Townsend and others suggests that adult children feel more responsibility for psychotic or senile parents than one might expect (Townsend, 1957 and 1962). Some workers interpret this devotion as simple love and family obligation, others as the product of anxiety and guilt. Whatever its source, the devotion is certainly there, though it does not mean that the home is necessarily a constructive place for a patient to be. The family may build their life around the patient's handicaps and delusions so that it becomes a little 'back ward' in the community.

The second major point is, what use does the family make of their informal network? One sometimes encounters statements in the literature that families with a psychotic patient are socially isolated (see for example Lomas, 1967). But often such isolation is treated as part of the pathogenic process, not as a response to the illness, and not as a possible combination of the two. Here again I should think more research and more open-mindedness would be helpful.

In this area I can do little more than ask questions, for I do not know of any research that has concentrated specifically on this problem, though social workers must know a lot about it and the current research of George Brown and his colleagues should shed light on it. Do the families of psychotic patients keep in touch with friends, neighbours, and relatives? Do they try to hide the psychosis from neighbours and friends but not from close relatives? Or do they close up entirely? Do they let close relatives help in some way to look after the patient? (Dr Scott assures me that in the families he studied, help of this sort was never sought.) Are relatives asked to help the family financially or with certain family tasks? Are there any systematic differences between families with highly connected networks and families with loose-knit networks in the use they make of their informal contacts? And what effect, direct or indirect, does the informal network have on the family's capacity to 'carry' a psychotic?

Finally, what of the formal network into which the family erupts when psychosis becomes manifest, a formal network that most ordinary families know nothing about? We who work in it know a lot about the formal structure of the mental health services. But how does it all look from the perspective of the family? I suspect it is quite a different picture. I think we need to know a lot more about what families do when they begin to suspect craziness in one of their members. Do they consult their general practitioner right away? And what does he do? Reassure them, give them drugs, send them to a psychiatric out-patient clinic? There have been studies of general practitioners' attitudes to psychiatric illness and psychiatric institutions, but to my mind such studies need to be linked up with simultaneous studies of the problem from the family's, the hospital's, and the local authority's perspective, before we have any real feel of how the system works.

Two points emerge about the family's relations to the formal network that deals with psychiatric crises. The first is that, in spite of all the talk about early diagnosis and treatment, families, general practitioners, and mental welfare officers are often reluctant to seek psychiatric help until the psychiatric crisis has become explosive. When the patient finally puts his brick through the window, everyone at last leaps into action. Why should this be so? In part it is because the patient, especially if he is paranoid, does not think he is ill and the family are terrified of disowning him and siding with 'them', the persecuting authorities. In the case of the general practitioner and the mental welfare officer, it is partly that if they cannot persuade the patient to go to hospital of his own accord, there is not much they can do until he *does* put a brick through a window. But there is another factor: going to hospital is often construed as failure by the general practitioner and the mental welfare officer. Success means keeping the patient in the community, failure means sending him to hospital – as if the hospital were the illness, not schizophrenia. Dennis Scott has tried to redefine the situation; failure is admission by psychiatric crisis; success is admission before psychiatric crisis. But it is an uphill struggle.

The second major point is that from the family's and the patient's point of view, the network of psychiatric services is quite extraordinarily split up and discontinuous. There is the general practitioner, the mental welfare officer, the admitting doctor, the ward doctor or doctors, the nursing staff, the hospital social worker, and possibly later on, another doctor at the out-patient clinic and perhaps a different social worker, not to mention clubs and various voluntary organizations that provide help. Psychotic patients have a tendency to project and 'lose' parts of themselves in their physical and social environment, so that both they and their families need an environment that is particularly straightforward and capable of holding them, in the sense of being a container that can keep the bits of the patient together until he finds himself again. It is difficult enough for normal people to cope with discontinuity. For a psychotic, with his precarious hold on his personal identity, real discontinuity in the external environment can be disastrous. Both psychiatric patients and their relatives are adept at exploiting, though usually not consciously, the available facilities for splitting and confusion – telling one thing to a nurse, something else to a doctor, something else to a psychiatric social worker, something else to a general practitioner, until everyone can get into a real muddle. On top of all this there is the constant pressure on beds, so great a pressure that often all the doctor and ward staff have time for is to put the patient on a sort of conveyor belt of tranquillizers and ward programmes and devote special attention only to patients that do not progress as expected.

What I am saying, in effect, is that I think psychiatric patients and their families would be better off if the formal psychiatric network were more highly connected. I doubt very much if such connectedness would greatly reduce the tendency towards admission by psychiatric crisis, however, for this tendency may well be an intrinsic part of the illness and the family constellation surrounding it. But greater connectedness in the formal network would cut down the numerous opportunities for communication failures and acting out. Anyone who has worked in this field knows that it is not easy to increase connectedness. There are formidable administrative and financial obstacles to be overcome as well as the usual professional jealousies and tendencies towards empire building (see especially Susser, 1962, for an analysis of the latter). Even when people consciously want to increase communication among themselves and continuity for patients, they sometimes develop unconscious or unspoken resistances to the changes they think or say they desire. At the same time I do not think one should assume that people will automatically resist every change; resistance depends on their conscious and unconscious perception of the relative advantages and disadvantages of the *status quo* compared to those of the proposed change.

One of the major administrative sources of disconnectedness is the tripartite division of the health service into the general practitioner service, the local authority health service, and the hospital service. The isolation of mental hospitals is another well known factor. I am sure you are all familiar with the several schemes afoot to overcome discontinuity: joint appointments and joint user arrangements between hospitals and local authorities, regrouping of subdivisions within hospitals so that each firm will provide in-patient and out-patient services for the patients and families of one geographical area; the establishment of psychiatric units in general hospitals – though that holds a gloomy future for the middle-and long-stay patients, and for the many imaginative schemes of social and industrial rehabilitation that have been developed in mental hospitals and that have not yet been successfully established in communities closer to the patients' homes.

In conclusion, the main point I wish to make is that to see the individual patient as a member of a family is not enough. The family belongs to a network, composed partly of informal contacts with friends, neighbours, and relatives, and partly of formal contacts with institutions and professions. The family is not isolated, but it is not *contained within* a community, except in the vague sense of the 'community' as a geographical or administrative area. The economic and ecological structure of our society make network formation inevitable, and network formation makes families generally vulnerable to stress. But we need to have a lot more systematic information about the way families use or avoid using both their informal and formal networks to cope with the various sorts of stress to which they are subjected.

REFERENCES

BALINT, M. & BALINT, E. (1961). *Psychotherapeutic techniques in medicine.* London: Tavistock Publications; Philadelphia: Lippincott.

BOTT, E. J. (1957). *Family and social network.* London: Tavistock Publications.

BROWN, G. W., *et al.* (1966). *Schizophrenia and social care.* Maudsley Monograph No. 17, London: Oxford University Press.

CAPLAN, G. (1961). *An approach to community mental health.* London: Tavistock Publications; New York: Grune & Stratton.

GOLDBERG, E. M. (1967). The family environment of schizophrenic patients. In Freeman, H. L. and Farndale, W. A. J. (eds.) *New aspects of the mental health services.* Oxford: Pergamon Press.

LAING, R. & ESTERSON, A. (1964). *Sanity, madness, and the family: the families of schizophrenics.* London: Tavistock Publications; New York: Basic Books.

LOMAS, P. (1967). The study of family relationships in contemporary society. In Lomas, P. (ed.), *The predicament of the family.* London: Hogarth.

MILLS, E. (1962). *Living with mental illness.* London: Routledge and Kegan Paul.

SEARLES, H. F. (1958). Positive feelings in the relationship between the schizophrenic and his mother. *Inter. J. Psycho-Anal.*, **39**, 569–86.

SCOTT, R. D. and ASHWORTH, P. A. (1965). The 'axis-value' and the transfer of psychosis. *Brit. J. med. Psychol.* **38**, 97–116.

SCOTT, R. D. and ASHWORTH, P. A. (1967). 'Closure' and the first schizophrenic breakdown. *Brit. J. med. Psychol.* **40**, 109–45.

SUSSER, M. W. (1962). Changing roles and co-ordination in mental health services. In *Sociological Review Monograph No. 5: Sociology and medicine*, pp. 61–90.

TOWNSEND, P. (1957). *The family life of old people.* London: Routledge and Kegan Paul.

—— (1962). *The last refuge: a survey of residential institutions and homes for the aged in England and Wales.* London: Routledge and Kegan Paul.

3 An Educational Perspective on Mental Health

BEN MORRIS

INTRODUCTION

I have chosen my text from the works of Sigmund Freud, from an essay, which deserves to be better known than it is, dealing with the educative interest of psychoanalysis and published in 1913. 'Only someone who can feel his way into the minds of children can be capable of educating them; and we grown-up people cannot understand children, because we no longer understand our own childhood' (Freud, 1951). We may like to think that the latter half of Freud's dictum is less true now than it was when he wrote it. For myself I always regard it as half a statement of fact and half a challenge to us as educators.

This fundamental insight of Freud's is of course only the beginning of wisdom in this field of mental health and education. Enlightened action nowadays requires that we take much more than this into account; but in the end, I think, we have again to turn to this initial insight as the essential clue to the direction our efforts should take.

If these opening words sound like the beginning of a sermon, I at least intend it to be a sermon in the modern manner, one shot through with a good deal of scepticism concerning the character of many of our cherished dogmas and beliefs both about mental health and about education. The sceptical edge to my own thinking derives from a number of sources. The first and most compelling is my own experience of the resistance exhibited by educational institutions towards the persistent attempts of many enlightened teachers to render their work more humane. A second is many years' reflection on the quasi-ideological character of a good deal of modern psychological thought, both academic and clinical. My approach also owes something to the efforts of modern

31

analytic philosophers to disentangle the intricate webs of *description* and moral *prescription* found in all mental health doctrines
and educational theories alike. Lastly I have been driven to
acknowledge the all-pervasive influence of culture on educative
practice, and of cultural conflicts within a changing society.

I am going to approach the fashioning of a perspective from
which to view the task of education in the development of a
mentally healthy community in three stages. In doing so I am
deliberately going to restrict my concern to so-called formal
education, in schools and colleges, while remaining aware, I hope,
that it is in the life of the family and the community at large that
the foundations must be laid. The first step it seems to me is to
establish a position from which a productive view of the relations
between education and mental health may be obtained. The
second step will be to examine some characteristic features of
current educational practice that seem, from the standpoint previously established, to be inimical to the interests of both mental
health and education. I want to look at these features of our
practice as expressing symptoms of *malaise* and so I hope finally
to devise some rationale for constructive endeavours in this field.
This last task might be (and in fact has been) styled the 'therapy of
education and educational institutions', but to use this language
would be, I think, to abandon the initial position about the
relation of mental health and education that I wish to establish.
Instead I propose to borrow a term from another language
altogether and to discuss the 'redemption' of our educational
enterprise.

I. MENTAL HEALTH AND EDUCATION

During this century it has gradually become obvious to us that
there is much common ground between the educational profession
on the one hand and other social professions, notably medicine,
psychology, and sociology, on the other. As in other instances,
however, the area in question seems more frequently to be viewed
as disputed territory rather than common ground. Myths and
mystiques grow fast on this fertile soil, and entrenched defensive
positions are rapidly taken up. These have served very greatly,
as is the nature of jungle growths, to obscure the actual features
of the territory itself, and there remain still to-day some fairly
genuine puzzles concerning what is at stake. I do not intend to

spend time on the myths and entrenched positions, save to remark that it seems to me that during my professional lifetime, medical omnipotence on the one hand, and educational paranoia on the other, have both notably diminished – a sign of a more healthy state of affairs.

Friendly and genuine co-operation is now much more the order of the day, but progress is still hindered by misconceptions on all sides, which although they ultimately have defensive roots do seem to some extent to be amenable to rational analysis. Thus many professional mental health workers, particularly medical ones, see education as essentially an affair of intellectual development, leaving emotional development in their care. Equally there are many educators who take essentially the same view. It is a highly convenient view for it appears to eliminate disputed territory. By the same token however it tends to eliminate common ground. A view which seems to me much more adequate in relation to all we know about human development is one that sees the concerns of mental health and education as having very substantial common interests.

Attempts to establish a middle position are common among those who are often styled 'progressive' educators, and many of them would claim the mental health of their pupils among their educational aims. This position is, however, often attacked from both sides, a common charge being that it confuses the roles of therapist and teacher. Other charges are that insufficient attention is in fact being given to mental health requirements, or that 'true' education is being neglected. Instructive examples of some current educational arguments will be found in the writings of one modern educational philosopher, Professor Richard Peters, who is himself notably friendly to, interested in, and knowledgeable about dynamic theories in psychology. One of Peters's notable contributions has been to clarify the notion of 'aims' in education by reaffirming the dependence of ends on means. By way of general illustration of this thesis he remarks, 'The Puritan and the Catholic both thought they were promoting God's Kingdom, but they thought it had to be promoted in a different manner. And the different manner made it quite a different Kingdom' (Peters, 1959). His work has served to remind educators, and we constantly need to be reminded of this, that it is *our educational practices* that in fact define our educational values. Incidentally this sauce for the educational goose is also sauce for the gander of mental health, and we might I think profit by examining what values are implied in current mental health practices.

Peters is interested in mental health but has some highly critical comments to make on the notion of 'mental health' as an educational aim, chiefly on the ground that it confuses the roles of therapist and teacher and reaffirms what he regards as the obnoxious notion that education must have an end beyond itself. Many of his remarks here are very apposite, but in the end I think he fails to follow his own prescriptions in relating ends to means; he does so primarily because he seems to me to underestimate the extent to which intellectual achievement and the very possibility of rationality itself (which he rightly regards as a cardinal human virtue) are intimately bound up with the ordering of the emotional life. For example, he thinks it important to remind teachers from time to time that their pupils have emotions to control, a love-life to lead, and a living to be earned. But he thinks this is better done by speaking of these things in terms of vocational training and of the training of the emotions and character, rather than in terms of mental health, which he sees as the province of the therapist. He regards it as a fact, and one to be deprecated, that a stress on mental health implies that 'children are to be treated as patients who have to be weaned in a kindly way to nibble at the raw meat of the modern world'. Since Peters's position is in many ways typical of an important current trend in educational thought, I propose to quote him at some length:

'It is unnecessary and misleading to saddle the teacher with a remedial function by saying that "mental health" should be one of his aims when what is covered by this term can be referred to in more traditional ways which do not carry the implication that the teacher is a special sort of doctor. This is not, of course, to say that there should not be experts readily available to whom the teacher can refer cases of breakdown; there are school doctors after all, and school dentists, so why not school psychiatrists? It is only to say that "mental health" should not be regarded as an aim of an educator.

'The cynic, of course, might reply that schools for many adolescents are in such a sorry state that there is little more that can be done than to have policemen in to stop riots, caretakers to keep the place clean, doctors and dentists to look after physical health and psychiatrically trained "teachers" to care for the "mental health" of the inmates. For the conditions of schooling and the attitudes of the inmates make any talk of "education" as out of place as a fashion parade would be on a dung-hill. But the cynic here concedes the main point which I am trying to make; and it is questionable whether his counsel of despair is justified in the light of examples of what can be done by imaginative teachers with the most unlikely material in appalling circumstances. Education is so much a matter of confidence, of imagination, and of enthusiasm; and it has not got to take the form of initiating farm-workers into a love for Shakespeare and symphony concerts. The emphasis on "mental health" reflects, among other things, a failure of nerve on the part of educators, a retreat from the positive' (Peters, 1964).

From this it seems to me that Peters has to make the distinctions he makes because he is using what I regard as inadequate concepts of mental health and of education.

It will now be apparent why the attempt rigidly to separate the concerns of education and mental health is so convenient. It is convenient for educators since it allows them to continue to treat human development as if it could be neatly divided into more or less independent segments: on the one hand the growth of intellect, on the other the training of the emotions and character. Any casualties that result from adopting such a view can then be handed over to the therapist. This has also been extremely convenient for, at any rate, the organization of mental health work in education. It leads to confining activity to the treatment of the casualties of the educational system and doing little about prevention. For what precisely would prevention really mean? Would it not mean in fact the redesigning of education in a way which allowed for the growth of persons as a whole? For thus might *some* of the casualties at any rate be prevented, those in which treating children as disembodied intellects or minds without passions and desires had played a large part. Of course the mental health professions have had numbers of pioneers who have seen the truth of all this and have tried to influence education in a radical way – just as there have been pioneers among educators who have tried to do much the same thing. But I think it not unfair to suggest that, by and large, this neat separation of tasks has served as a defensive device against more radical approaches. It has allowed the teacher to remain in his classroom undisturbed by radical doubts, and has allowed diagnosticians and therapists to get on with their specifically clinical work. Some of my pioneering friends in child psychiatry and in educational psychology are likely to protest that this is unfair and that the real resistance to more radical approaches is in the schools. There is plenty of resistance there of course, but does it exist only there?

This discussion raises the question of the nature of modern concepts of *mental health* and of *education* and whether the major values implicit in these concepts are ones that can be shared. We are now, I think, growing out of the notion of mental health as implying the absence of conflict within the personality. This was once quite widely regarded as its most important internal criterion. Correlative with this was the notion that mental health implied 'adjustment' to the social *mores* by means of conformity to them. Modern ideas, I think, centre on two rather different notions. Health is first of all demonstrated by a developed capacity to deal with both internal conflict and external stress, through containing them, and growing both through them and by means of them. It is thus demonstrated in the capacity, as Freud put it, to both love and work effectively, in the widest senses of both these terms; and this would, I venture to think, include all that Peters wants to safeguard within education itself.

Secondly, to love and work effectively implies the capacity of the individual to come to terms with social demands in a way that means he is not simply a conforming victim of social pressures but can make his own distinctive contribution to society, however small. Implicit in these newer conceptions is the idea of human beings as persons, each enjoying some degree of autonomy, an autonomy expressed in terms of internal integration and limited by the similar autonomy of others. The relative nature of this conception of mental health is obvious, but we are by no means lacking in practical criteria in terms of which we may say that persons enjoy good or poor mental health!

What about our conceptions of education? I see the roles of educator and therapist as distinct, and as conditioned by their different settings and skills; but I also see them as closely related and as needing to influence one another. To have a clear conception of each it is necessary to have an understanding of what they have in common as well as of what makes them different. It is the communality with which I am here concerned. Foremost among the things they have in common is a concern for the effective functioning of human beings as persons in a civilized community. To be concerned with this as educators is not, in my view, to subscribe uncritically to what is often pejoratively labelled (particularly now in the USA) as 'soft pedagogy'. On the contrary it demands an understanding both of the delicacy and complexity, *and* of the robustness and simplicity, of human functioning, and an understanding of the intimate relations between emotional and intellectual growth and between the personal and the impersonal aspects of experience. Moreover such understanding has to issue in procedures that take account of stabilities and instabilities, of weaknesses and strengths, and of the conditions *for* and implications *of* success and failure in learning. The essential common task of educator and therapist is one, I think, we may define as promoting both personal and social well-being, and such well-being is at present impossible for most people in our kind of society without adequate achievements in the sphere of both love and work.

We may conclude then by asserting that educators and mental health workers have vital interests in common in nourishing stability in the young and in making possible genuine personal achievements. But to do this teachers must often be concerned to reduce, and if possible eliminate, sources of unnecessary conflict in the lives of children and young people. To talk of 'unnecessary' conflicts is of course to beg a number of very large and important questions, but examples of what I mean are easily found. To demand of children the successful accomplishment of tasks that are quite beyond them, in terms of their experience, resources, and situation at any given time, is to subject them to quite unnecessary and often highly damaging conflicts. Our educational institutions continually make such demands on very large numbers of children.

Yet more is required of teachers than the reduction of unnecessary conflicts. They have to enable children to tolerate necessary conflicts and tensions and, in attempting to do this, what is crucial is the quality of their relationships with their pupils. The notion of *discipline* so dear to the heart of teachers is one that at once

D

enshrines and obscures the essential character of productive relations between teachers and taught. The discipline which matters is one that is directed towards the growth of *internal controls* in the young, that will sustain them in conflicts of feeling, while not demanding crippling sacrifices in the expression of natural desires, interests, and talents. Yet to do this effectively within institutions that are *based on quite other notions of discipline* seems, at present, largely to be beyond all but the most gifted of teachers. To understand our failures here, we must turn to some of the major features of our current practices that exhibit an unmistakable *malaise*.

2. A CRITIQUE OF EDUCATIONAL PRACTICE

It is, of course, easy to cite the presenting symptoms of mental ill health in the educational system in terms of the relatively large number of individual problems thrown up in schools and colleges, *not*, as estimated simply by official figures for maladjustment, serious mental illness, or crime, *but* as known personally to many teachers and parents. We might also cite the relatively low morale of the teaching profession, which has a poor image, and tends to be preoccupied with status, pay, and internal and external scapegoating.

To offer a fair critique of current educational practice that would illumine this situation is more difficult. It is necessary, I think, to take account of the fact that there are many changes going on and that 'enlightened' theoretical views are greatly to the fore in academic circles. Thus, in the higher echelons of the academic educational world, i.e. in teacher education, accepted doctrines include an emphasis on the growth of children as whole persons, the close interrelation of maturation and nurture, the importance of readiness, of developmental sequences, and of meaningful activity in learning, of the role of play and creative expression, and of the enormous significance of individual differences in capacities, temperaments, and interests, and of individually adjusted goals. Yet in the schools themselves, although there are notable developments in many infant and in some junior schools, these principles are acknowledged more in the breach than in the observance. Why?

Two major factors seem to be at work. First there is the enormous expansion of educational provision that has taken place in the last fifty years, an expansion accompanied by a heightened struggle for higher social status and other social rewards, and one that has latterly taken place in an era of acute teacher shortage. Inevitably in this situation conflicts of value have set in, as the result of changing ways of life and of the inclusion in the upper reaches of education of large sections of the population that were relatively little influenced by it in the past. These factors will probably be fairly prominent features of our educational and social scene for some time to come, and they are outside the direct control of the educational system, although influencing it decisively.

The second factor is again one that seems to me to be endemic in the educational situation itself, namely the tension between the generations crystallized within the schools in terms of pupils and their parents on one side and teachers on the other, and between older and newer conceptions of education among teachers themselves. Largely as a result of these two factors we find that schools as institutions show very high resistance to change. It is precisely here, it seems to me, that we ought to focus our attention most firmly; for in the light of modern psychological and sociological knowledge it does seem possible that we could induce much more rapid change, which would produce a better balance between external pressures and the response of the school system, and a lessening of destructive tension between the generations. It is therefore reasonable to suppose that an examination of some of the major symptoms of educational *malaise* might help to focus our efforts on crucial areas in which more rapid change might be possible. A list of such educational ills makes dull or exciting reading depending on one's temperament. They are meat and drink to educational radicals bent mainly on denunciation, and to mental health workers who have not seriously envisaged what changing an educational system entails. What follows here is not intended as destructive criticism, but purely as a symptomatology of a system urgently in need of constructive measures of help.

I would begin with the still largely adult-centred nature of our school curricula, which persists throughout the system, despite splendid pioneering work in those of our infant, junior, and secondary modern schools that have gone over to learner-centred approaches. The orthodox curriculum is often apparently effective in the short term, but its long term inefficiency for all but the ablest children is scarcely in doubt. This stress on *immediate efficiency* rather than on the development of long term competencies is, moreover, exercised over a narrow range of accomplishments, resulting for many children in serious deprivation of social, scientific, and aesthetic experience, and providing little or no experience of co-operative learning in groups or of mutual help. The standards exacted reflect a stress on average attainments rather than on individual goals; that is, statistical averages of performance are used as mandatory norms for individuals. It is true of course that in many areas where the tyranny of the 11+ has been diminished through the development of forms of comprehensive secondary education, the primary schools are beginning to emerge from servitude and from the winter of their discontent. Spring is in the air, even if scarcely noticeable in far too many quarters. The Plowden Report has been heartening in this respect, yet it pointed to the existence of large areas of social and educational deprivation.

The secondary system is at present disrupted by often ill-conceived and over-hasty reorganization. There are, of course, some surprisingly fine comprehensive schools; and there can be little doubt that this sort of organization has come to stay, and that it can be made to work reasonably well, if only we take time to plan the change and understand the special human problems of large units and of the diverse social backgrounds of the pupils. But the distinctive features of the secondary system, responsible for its major ills, remain, *whatever the form of organization.* There are three main features. The first, which now directly affects perhaps sixty or more per cent of children, and indirectly affects the others, is the rigid external, competitive, and highly selective examination system, which is closely linked to the social pressures in our society. The total effect of this examination system, from which few escape undamaged, is again a narrowing of experience, anxiety based on adult pressure and expectation, the experience by many of failure at quite an early age, unsound achievements based on mechanical skills, and highly practised verbal responses without adequate understanding.

The second feature, which affects mainly the less able half of the pupils, is the failure to engage them meaningfully in their own education and to give them any adequate vocational aspirations and preparation. This is what is now known as the Newsom problem, the problem of adolescents forced to remain in schools that take little or no account of their genuine needs, interests, and talents.

The third feature affects all in some measure and is characterized by the prevalence of systems of control based largely on adult-imposed discipline, as opposed to discipline arising from tasks and mediated by working groups. These controls are related primarily to adult conveniences and adult maladjustment, and there is little or no insight into unconscious adult complicity in producing undesirable behaviour. The result is, of course, both over- and under-development of internal controls in pupils, and a relative failure to develop deep interests in activities and achievements for their own sake as distinct from an interest based on examination results. There is continual conflict between pupils, parents, and school authorities over petty restrictions concerning dress and appearance and over unimportant offences. Relatively little use is made of adolescent idealism and desire for genuine responsibility. At the deepest level we are dealing here with our failure to understand the effects of prolonging social immaturity after the onset of physical sex maturity. While the great majority of so-called teenage behaviour problems are not just teenage problems, but are problems resulting from inappropriate adult responses, our preoccupation with them prevents a proper understanding of the real and to some extent inevitable problems about authority, independence, and sexual behaviour that all adolescents have to face in our changing society.

What can be done about all this? Nowadays we do not look for panaceas, nor if we are wise do we dream of educational utopias, but rather we are concerned to look for ways in which beneficial changes may gradually be introduced into the system. I shall limit myself to two examples of what I think can be done, and in each case it will be apparent that everything depends on being able to bring about in those most concerned changes in their attitudes *to their own problems*.

3. THE REDEMPTION OF THE EDUCATIONAL ENTERPRISE

How can the educational system set about redeeming itself, at least in part? I would like to illustrate the possibilities by referring to two areas in which something is already being done.

(a) *The Examination System*

The real evils here do not stem from what is often called the social rat-race, nor from the necessary differentiation among the life paths of individuals according to their talents and the needs of society. These are permanent features of our culture. So long as we simply condemn examinations or regard them as necessary evils, we can take no practical steps towards a critical diagnosis. Critical studies have, however, been made and the way forward is now known in principle and, in a small way, in practice. The essential, and in principle remediable, evils of our examination systems are their *externality* to the work of teaching. 'Exams' control teaching, and this is the reverse of what should be the case. There is now apparent, through the work of the Schools Council and other agencies, a move to replace external examinations by internal examinations externally moderated. This choice is now open to all schools entering pupils for the Certificate of Secondary Education. We are not surprised, of course, that only a relatively few schools and teachers wish to avail themselves of this freedom. Such freedom is not easily welcomed because it entails new responsibility, and the rethinking of current practices. External examinations are a defensive prop for the majority of teachers, whose own training and experience have not prepared them for the responsibilities of deciding what shall be taught, how it shall be taught, and of making their own assessments, even if externally checked.

Of course, a system of internal examinations only gives us a point of entry. But it is an essential one. The major task now is to prepare teachers, both new and experienced, for an entirely fresh conception of their responsibilities. Few teachers at the moment command the necessary skills or confidence. Considering the low public esteem of the profession and its poor rewards we cannot expect immediate enthusiasm. But there are signs of change, and university institutes of education, teachers' colleges, and local education authorities now have opportunities to do something about the situation. The re-education of serving teachers is now showing signs of becoming an extremely important branch of our work. Essentially the approach must be one in which teachers themselves, under guidance, are enabled to rethink and re-equip themselves. The inducing of important changes in attitudes is of course essential to this process.

(b) *The Reform of the Secondary Curriculum*

Turning now to a second major area of *malaise*, the unsuitability of schools, as they exist, as places in which young persons can grow to maturity, we also find that important new moves are afoot, again with the Schools Council in the role of promoting agency. The problem is at its most acute, of course, in the socially underprivileged areas, but with the coming of comprehensive schooling it affects all areas. If we bear in mind here also the major conflicts between the generations, between youthful needs and adult attitudes, we may see the problem as an entirely general one.

The new moves again centre on the re-education of serving teachers, priority being given to those from the socially and educationally underprivileged sectors. The problems to be tackled here are even more far-reaching than in the reform of the examination system, since they centre on strongly held beliefs and attitudes having their origins in teachers' own childhoods. Again startling advances are not to be expected, and we need to give a great deal more thought than we have done to the central role of psychological and sociological studies in teacher education. It is to this theme that I finally want to turn. As I see it the problem is essentially one of helping others to acquire some of the art of human understanding, and at the same time perchance to deepen one's own.

4. TEACHING THE ART OF HUMAN UNDERSTANDING

Teachers of course vary enormously in this essential quality. Some, perhaps by nature but certainly by upbringing, have it in generous measure; others are almost, one is tempted to think, without it. Yet experience shows that most students and teachers can augment their powers of insight, imagination, and sympathy through properly conceived courses of study, containing both practical and theoretical elements. Here psychology as an aid to educational thinking faces its crucial test, and in my view at present very largely fails. It tends to fail for a number of reasons. Among these is the quite common assumption that the beginner should be introduced to such studies in the form of a rigorous scientific discipline, with an almost purely experimental or technological basis. It follows that such an approach virtually rules out any significant self-reference. Instead of being encouraged to reflect on his own real experiences of personal interaction, the student is carefully steered clear of any such alarming reflections by being presented with purely objective studies. Instead of augmenting students' powers of understanding, very often such powers as they may have are actually reduced, by measures that act as additional defences against self-knowledge. A common accompaniment of such studies is a subtle indoctrination in a scientific ideology that ignores or plays down any conception of human beings as persons, and indeed replaces such a conception by one in which men, women, and particularly children are merely responding organisms to be helpfully manipulated through scientific understanding based on a behaviourist model.

Clearly, if changes in behaviour are, as far as possible, to be self-induced and to result in a deeper understanding of personality and interpersonal relations, then psychological studies must have quite a different orientation. They must begin from a view of psychology that sees it as a mode of study and reflection based on the realities of interpersonal experience, and augmented as necessary through controlled and objective studies. The conduct of and the settings for such study are important, and no course of lectures on modern theories of personality is adequate for this purpose. Moreover, within the setting of the professional education of teachers, any direct attack on the personal problems of teachers is bound to fail. Group settings are essential, and the most relevant material is that which the students and teachers can themselves provide from their own experience. It is in such a setting, in which the focus of attention is on the professional tasks, roles, and problems of teachers and schools, that the participants most easily begin to gain understanding of the subtle interweaving of intellectual and emotional problems and of the influences of childhood experiences on developed adult attitudes. Understanding is gained too of the sources and nature of tensions within schools as institutions, and of how these might be reduced. In particular, courses for heads of schools that make use of their own familiar problems as a basis of discussion are an important new development.

Here I return to the original quotation from Freud. The understanding of childhood and youth is in principle the understanding of one's own past, and of the way this past lives on in the present, continually colouring and helping to shape responses to others here and now, and particularly responses to children and young people. We must not of course expect too much in the way of change to result from such insightful study. But if glimpses can be obtained, and held, of the role of anxiety, hostility, guilt, and love in shaping our professional and institutional behaviour, much has been done.

Although to know, and actively to be able to feel, what it is like to be young, while remaining adult oneself, lies at the heart of the problems of education, it is by itself no sufficient means of redemption, but it is an indispensable basis for any significant attempts to redeem the educational enterprise. I have had to omit much in this brief perspective, in particular, the importance of expanding the roles of clinically trained educational psychologists, and of promoting the introduction of the newer professional cadre of school counsellors. Clearly the need for the variety of leadership roles played by psychiatrists, psychologists, social workers, and school counsellors is great, but the essential job will always lie in helping the 'general practitioners' in the schools to a fuller understanding of themselves and of what they are doing in educating children.

The tasks facing us are of course immense. How could they be otherwise? But to gain a wider acceptance of the way in which mental health concepts can enrich our view of education, and so enable education to play a fuller part in promoting a healthier society, would be in itself an important advance. I see no reason for despair. In sombre moments one sometimes entertains Samuel Beckett's wry comment that 'Life is a syndrome which admits of no palliation', but despite its kernel of seeming wisdom, one knows this to be untrue. One has only to visit some of the pioneering schools within our state system and participate with the children in their activities to know that a great deal of palliation is possible, and also to feel that *one* essential clue to the redemption of much of human life lies here. I therefore prefer Edwin Muir's vision to Samuel Beckett's.

> *One foot in Eden still, I stand*
> *And look across the other land.*
> *The world's great day is growing late,*
> *Yet strange these fields that we have planted*

So long with crops of love and hate.
Time's handiworks by time are haunted,
And nothing now can separate
The corn and tares compactly grown.
The armorial weed in stillness bound
About the stalk; these are our own.
Evil and good stand thick around
In the fields of charity and sin
Where we shall lead our harvest in.

Yet still from Eden springs the root
As clean as on the starting day.

EDWIN MUIR[1]

REFERENCES

FREUD, S. (1951). The claims of psychoanalysis to scientific interest –
(H) The educative interest. *Complete Works Standard English Edition*,
vol. 13, p. 189. London: Hogarth Press.

MUIR, EDWIN (1960). *Collected poems*. London: Faber and Faber.

PETERS, R. S. (1959). *Authority, responsibility, and education*. London:
Allen & Unwin.

PETERS, R. S. (1964). 'Mental health' as an educational aim. *Stud.*
Philos. Educat., **3**, 197.

© Ben Morris, 1971

[1] From *Collected Poems* (Faber & Faber, 1960). Reprinted by kind per-
mission of the publishers.

4 Social Institutions and Individual Adjustment

ELLIOTT JAQUES

I

It has long been assumed – and surely with some reason – that the society in which we live affects our behaviour and our mental well-being. But the actual nature of this connexion between the individual and his society has been difficult to establish – and it is not clear yet whether we can determine that connexion with any exactitude. During the past twenty years, however, very considerable advances have been made in detailed exploration of this problem. These advances have a not inconsiderable importance for psychiatry and for the general alleviation of mental disorder and stress.

In particular, I would like to illustrate the kind of evidence now becoming available in the following main areas:

(a) the possible connexion between social structure and mental illness – in particular, the significance of differences in the incidence of various types of mental illness in different social classes;
(b) the effects upon the behaviour of individuals and the stresses to which they are subjected, of the social institutions, organization, and groups of which they are members;
(c) the implications of these findings for the organization of psychiatric hospitals for treatment; and
(d) the development of healthy social institutions – that is to say, institutions that are organized so as to minimize unnecessary stress upon individuals.

I shall use the phrase requisite organization to refer to the healthy type of organization – requisite in the sense of conforming

47

both to the individual and to the institutional requirements of the situation.

II

The most obvious connexion between social relationships and mental illness is to be seen in the family. Psychodynamic studies show up sharply the impact, for example, of the mother's behaviour upon the mental development of the child. We know the effects upon infant development when these relationships go astray – through neglect by the mother, or through the emotional incapacity of the parents to cope with the demands of the child by providing adequate love and security or by taking and coping with the child's hate and aggression.

I do not propose to dwell upon these family relationships, however, in this paper. I do not propose to do so for one main reason, a reason that may help to outline more precisely the nature of my object. For, even though it may be the case that families and their behaviour affect – and seriously affect – the mental development of their members, it is equally the case that improving the mental climate within families is not much easier than improving the mental health of the individual.

Psychological treatment of individuals, and of families, is a profoundly important endeavour – for the individual, for the family, for knowledge, and for society. But this type of work, as we are all well aware, pecks only at the fringe of the problem of mental illness from society's point of view. We must provide treatment for willing individuals and for willing families, but doing so does not relieve the mass of illness and emotional stress that exists all around us. To tackle this larger-scale problem, methods that are larger in scope and in scale are required.

Educational methods are usually the first to be thought of, when we talk about mental health programmes on any scale. I am going to suggest that educational programmes are notoriously ineffective when it comes to changing behaviour. In doing so, I am not taking up a pessimistic theme. For I wish to go further, and to suggest that we may be able to grasp this large-scale problem, and to reduce it significantly, by paying adequate attention to the organization of our society and of the institutions within our society. This particular path is not an easy one. There are great technical obstacles in the way – we must, in the first place, extend our knowledge of what makes requisite institutions, far beyond what we presently know. And, even if we knew more, there are always powerful forces and resistances counterpoised against change. But given the development of the required knowledge, our society and general social institutions – unlike the family – are amenable to conscious organization and control by means of agreed policies. We can decide how we are going to organize them, and do it. We can thereby lay the foundation for tangible and significant changes in individual behaviour, not by exhortation or hopeful education, but by the practical and explicable step of changing the setting in which each one behaves.

I am going to suggest, therefore, that attention to our social institutions and the way they are organized and administered, is an essential, practical, hard-headed exercise in community mental health – that sound organization and administration of our institutions is an essential component for the improvement of mental health.

III

Let me first of all introduce my theme from my own personal experience, an experience that may serve to explain why, as a practising psychoanalyst dealing with the unconscious fantasy life of adults and children, I am also so deeply concerned with the social reality within which we live. For exactly twenty years now, I have been engaged roughly half-time in a social consultancy role to an engineering company – the Glacier Metal Company – on what has come to be known as the Glacier Project. My relationship with the firm may be familiar to you, since it was patterned upon the type of relationship that is usual in medical research. The project began in 1948 when I was at the Tavistock Institute, financed by a Government research grant, and has continued from 1951 to the present financed by the Company itself. The work has been carried out in collaboration with the Company in the sense that my services have been available to any individuals or groups in the Company who wish to seek them. It is my task to help them to analyse the nature of their problems, and not to make recommendations as to what they ought to do. The work that has gone on, therefore, has been initiated from within the Company. The model used has been that of clinical research in psychological medicine, where, as you know, one of the main problems is to gain access to data. What we did was to set up an independent role in the firm in which access was obtained as a result of the invitation to help with various ongoing problems.

Within this independent relationship, I worked in nearly every area of organization and management, including, for example, the development of a Works Council structure and legislative functions; the total field of executive organization; the representative system, including trade-union relations; level-of-work measurement, payment structure, and individual progress; appeals procedures; company policy and management training; economic, accountancy, sales, and research organization; and so on.

It has been possible for me in the course of this project not only to help to effect gross changes in organization, but also to be on the spot, and involved in follow-up work in connexion with these changes for periods of years afterwards. I have thus had the opportunity to observe what happened to individuals as a result of these changes. What has impressed me is the radical nature of the changes in behaviour of many individuals. It is not all black and white. But by and large there is an easier atmosphere.

Let me illustrate the kind of problem that arose, and the sort of outcome that was achieved.

A works manager was in charge of a factory employing about a thousand people. He was supposed to be responsible for the quantity and quality of the work turned out, and for seeing that it was completed on schedule, all within the various limitations imposed upon him by his equipment and tooling, the quality and availability of supplies, the efficacy of permitted methods, and the quality of the labour to hand. The apparent extent of his responsibility showed him completely in charge.

The actual situation, once you looked beneath the surface, was quite different. The general manager to whom the works manager was responsible had a number of other direct subordinates: a chief production engineer in charge of methods, a chief production controller in charge of scheduling and deliveries, a chief inspector responsible for quality, a chief accountant, a personnel manager, and a chief buyer. Each of these had a considerable staff under him with duties that took them on to the shop floor in contact with the works manager's command at several levels removed.

What actually took place at supervisory and operating levels? Methods engineers, layout engineers, time-study engineers fixed and altered methods and times and did development work; scheduling officers responsible to the chief production controller routed work, loaded machines, and revised schedules as required; and, without going into detail, the staffs of the chief inspector, chief accountant, personnel manager, and chief buyer also had their duties to carry out at shop-floor level. In fact (the actual situation), the production managers shared responsibility for methods with the production engineers, for delivery with the production controllers, for quality with the inspectors, and so forth.

Now move back to the works manager. He was by-passed by a network of instructions from these specialist colleagues to his subordinates not at all under his own control. He could be said to be in charge of production – except for methods, quality, cost, delivery, personnel, and budgets! Was he in fact in charge of his factory, as was theoretically the case? The answer is, clearly, no!

You may believe that this example of inconsistency between the theoretical and the actual situations is a special one. That is not so. This particular example is a common pattern of organization in industry, and one that is the cause of a great deal of stress and inefficiency. In the instance given, the effect was frustration, accompanied by susceptibility to fatigue and a chronic sense of overwork, in a series of four works managers who succeeded each other in the job over a period of eight years. Moreover, the people carrying responsibility in the specialist positions I have described were similarly affected.

An extensive analysis of the work situation led to the recognition that the requisite organization demanded by the type of work carried in the works manager role was different from either the theoretical or the actual. By requisite organization, I mean the establishment of jobs with stated responsibilities assigned to colleague positions. Examination of the underlying situation showed that the role of works manager needed to be taken out of the direct line of command, and explicitly established as an administrative position. The shops were reorganized into units of 200–400 operators, divided into sections of 10–50 members under a section manager. Each unit manager had his own specialist staff of production engineers and production controllers, allocated to him, and was given his own personnel specialist. The net effect has been an organization in which responsibility and authority are not out of line with each other, as was previously the case.

It is not my purpose to go into details of this new organization. The point to emphasize, however, is that it was built up in relation to the work to be done, the essential principle being that of building an organization and establishing mechanisms whereby members actually were accountable for what they were stated to be, in the sense of their responsibilities being consistent with each other, and of their having the authority that goes with the responsibilities for which they may be called to account.

The effect of the change upon individuals – and I have been able to observe it for over three years now – has been to increase decisiveness. Complaints about fatigue due to overlapping responsibilities have correspondingly diminished – diminished, that is, in all but a few instances of individuals who had been enabled to play out neuroses in the previous situation, and who now had to find other ways to deal with their personal disturbances.

Production controllers no longer have to beat their way around the shops, using the 'iron fist in the velvet glove' to fulfil a responsibility for which they had not been given the requisite authority. The methods engineers are no longer treated as outsiders, the 'strangers from upstairs'. And it is possible for operational managers realistically to be held accountable for their work.

In similar vein, requisite institutions have been developed which allow for all employees at all levels to interact through elected representatives with the managing director, in agreeing or modifying the policies governing their individual duties and entitlements. The methods are not in terms of irrelevant concepts of industrial democracy, or of group decision, but of social institutions that take into account the actualities of the power situation, and therefore can succeed in mediating power. Every employee also has the absolute right of appeal against any decision of his manager that affects him. The effect of these institutions on the outlook and behaviour of both managers and militant representatives has been dramatic. Industrial tension has been markedly reduced. As managers, shop stewards, and staff representatives put it, they have explicit and agreed constitutional means for resolving disputes. It is not that they do not have arguments. But they have more telling and fruitful arguments.

And the arguments can take place when the problem occurs, rather than simmering under cover, combining with other unresolved stresses, and eventually erupting with a bang. These constitutional procedures were developed out of social analyses and modifications conducted from 1948 to 1955. They have been fairly stable for the past twelve years, despite considerable changes in personnel, and are therefore, I would say, entitled to be thought of as pretty fairly tested.

I believe that we have even discovered a fundamental solution to the vexed national problem of arranging for equitable payment – that is to say, payment related to the level of responsibility that a person is called upon to carry. If that is true, and I think we have got far enough at least to demonstrate that the problem is resolvable, then think how much social tension based upon economic rivalry, envy, jealousy, suspicion, and class hatred might be alleviated!

Requisite social organization and procedures related to the realities of the social situation, as revealed by analysis, can provide a setting for gross behavioural change. That is the lesson for me from the Glacier Project. But the question still remains, how far can it be said that these changes in behaviour are connected with improvements in mental health? Do they, for instance, lead to changes in family relationships that are conducive to mentally healthy atmospheres? My data here fall far short of what one would like to know. But I would like to turn to evidence from another research project that does suggest that what happens at the work place may in fact profoundly affect marital and family relationships for the better or for the worse.

IV

In a study of families and work in the Detroit area, Miller and Swanson (1958) have shown how the switch from an entrepreneurial situation to a bureaucratic situation by the head of the family can have radical effects upon the patterns of individual relationships within the family. When the father works in an entrepreneurial role, his own concern for resources and for the people he serves so affects his own outlook that he inculcates into the family the *mores* that are usually thought of as the 'protestant ethic'. When the father is employed, however, in the relative security of a bureaucratic situation, when he himself no longer

risks personal loss as the result of his decisions, a loosening of
his concern for others and for resources occurs, with a consequent loosening of the moral standards that he inculcates in
the family, and an increase in social deviance and emotional disturbance. Interactions between individual behaviour and social
setting of the kind teased out in the Miller and Swanson study
require to be carried out much more extensively if we are to
be able to help society organize its affairs on a more rational
basis.

v

The Miller and Swanson study gives some idea of the significance
of the results that can be obtained from carefully conducted large-
scale social analyses. Such studies have become more frequent
recently in the field of epidemiology of mental illness, and some
data from that area can help to extend our present analysis of the
interaction between the individual and his social environment to
the level of society as a whole.

For many years now, it has been assumed that the more severe
mental illnesses occurred among the most economically and
socially distressed sections of our urban populations. This
assumed relationship has been established fairly conclusively in
a series of studies, notably in the United States. During the 1950s
in Chicago, for instance, Faris and Dunham (1965) showed that
schizophrenia was significantly more frequent among the working classes, and depressive illness more frequent among the
middle classes. It might be argued, of course, that such studies
merely demonstrate that schizophrenics and schizophrenic families fall to the bottom of the social scale and there reproduce
themselves. But that this explanation is perhaps too simple was
suggested by a unique feature of the follow-up study.

The social structure of Chicago is peculiarly related to its
geography. The city is like a great half-circle with its straight
side stretching along the waterfront of Lake Michigan. It was
populated by successive waves of immigrants, each landing and
settling first in the 'Loop', the central area of the city, at the waterfront. As each new wave of immigrants came in, the earlier
arrivals, now prospering, moved outwards to form concentric
semicircles around the Loop. Thus as time went by, the city came
to be composed of different ethnic groups, situated in a series of

concentric bands with the Loop at their centre, with the groups becoming increasingly prosperous the farther one went from the centre of the city.

A sample from the ethnic groups in each of these concentric bands again showed that schizophrenia was significantly more frequent in the Loop, and became less frequent as one moved into the more prosperous outlying areas. That is to say, as each ethnic group adapted, and became more prosperous, the incidence of schizophrenia decreased.

These findings were more recently duplicated, on a much larger scale, by Hollingshead and Redlich (1958) in New Haven, Connecticut. There the population of one district of the city, called Yorkville, was studied *in toto*. Every family was investigated psychiatrically. The findings were in many respects startling; for example, some 25 per cent of the population were assessed as being urgently in need of psychiatric treatment. For our present interest, the finding was again clear: namely, that schizophrenia was an illness that occurred to a significantly higher degree among working-class families, while depression and neurosis had a relatively higher incidence among middle-class families.

These studies, and related findings, strongly suggest that poor economic circumstances, in modern industrial urban conditions, are conducive of severe psychiatric disturbance of a schizophrenic character. What might be the reason? The most likely explanation, in my view, that has been propounded, is the simple neglect that can and does occur in urban poverty – not necessarily lack of love, but the physical neglect of infants and children because their mothers are working or financially harassed. Not that all working-class mothers neglect their children, but consistent emotional and physiological care is not so readily possible under conditions of crowded working-class family life and facilities, so often made worse by economic uncertainty and despair.

Our presumptive conclusion, therefore, is that there is increasing evidence from epidemiological studies that improved economic conditions in urban industrial society may in time reduce the incidence of the more severe forms of mental illness, such as schizophrenia, because of the effect upon the structure and content of relationships within families.

VI

I have tried to illustrate some connexions between social organization and behaviour – moving from the micro-social region of
industrial work, through the relation between work and family
life, to the impact of the macro-social structure upon human
relations and emotional development. These considerations, it
may be apparent, might have implications that are very close to
home for those of us who are concerned with the care and treatment of psychiatric patients in mental hospitals. For hospital
organization itself may, and does, suffer from some of the same
obscurities in organization that are found in industry. To take an
equivalent problem to that of the works manager I described
earlier: Who is accountable for the effective running of a hospital?
What is the authority of the consultants? of the nurses? of the
administrators? And for what are they held accountable? And by
whom? And what are the criteria of assessment? These questions
do not have ready and easy answers.

   But it may also be asked if it really matters whether or not the
authority and accountability, the organization and administration,
are all that explicit. The answer to that question is really fairly
clear. For example the Stanton and Schwarz (1954) studies
describe vividly the manipulations that are open to disturbed
patients when the relationships between doctors and nurses are
confused by lack of explicitness about how far the responsibility
and authority of each extends. The attendant stresses in the professional sphere may be capitalized on by patients, not always to
their betterment.

   We have a long way to go in sorting out the optimum organizational requirements of all hospitals, including mental hospitals.
It is likely to be a difficult task, since hospitals, with their multi-
plicity of interacting professional and administrative groups, are
among the most complex of social institutions. But the problem
has begun to be tackled, and when optimum types of organization
have been formulated, I believe that a major contribution will
have been made to mental hospital treatment.

VII

In general terms then, the problem of mental illness must be
tackled on many fronts: individual treatment; treatment of fami-

lies; educational programmes; and the elucidation and establishment of requisite social institutions to provide a supportive social frame within which sound behaviour patterns can be encouraged and reinforced. Widespread mental health calls for a healthy social surrounding. But, in fact, society is in turmoil and still has to learn to live in large groups. We are only at the beginning of an understanding of how individuals interact with each other and with their broader social environment.

The nature of a healthy society and requisite social institutions tends to be a matter for political debate. As human scientists, we can no longer let the matter rest there. Psychiatric and social research combined may have much to say about how society ought to organize itself, in terms of the requirements of the mental life of the individual, upon which ultimately the good of that society will depend. In short, it is to be hoped that we are entering an era in which social policy and organization will be determined not by political debate and negotiation alone, but by political debate informed and reinforced by hard findings, concepts, and formulations from research into the actualities of the relationship between the individual and the social institutions he inhabits.

REFERENCES

FARIS, R. E. L. & DUNHAM, H. W. (1965). *Mental Disorders in urban areas.* Chicago: University of Chicago Press.

HOLLINGSHEAD, A. B. & REDLICH, F. C. (1958). *Social class and mental illness.* New York: Wiley.

MILLER, D. R. & SWANSON, G. E. (1958). *The changing American parent.* New York: Wiley.

STANTON, & SCHWARZ, M. S. (1954). *The mental hospital.* New York: Basic Books.

5 The Changing Role of the Psychotherapist

Leopold Bellak (1964), refers to community psychiatry as the third revolution in psychiatry. He adds, however, that what this term covers is not so much a revolution in psychiatric thought as a new phase – one that has evolved under the impact of many developments, in particular psychoanalysis, the social services, and the acquisition of powerful drugs for the modification of disturbed behaviour. The various kinds of activities within this overall endeavour are closely linked and there have inevitably been looseness and overlapping in the terms used to describe them. There appears now to be some agreement about terms and I should like to state briefly the usage that I shall adopt.

Community mental health embraces both overall goals and the programmes of action required to attain them. A first goal, shared with medicine in general, is prevention, i.e. the elimination of the causes of mental illness and the maintenance of this prophylactic endeavour. As with physical well-being, this goal must be complemented by the more positive aim of creating the conditions for 'the optimum performance of human beings as civilized creatures' (Gregg, 1944). As the same author continues, the pursuit of this goal 'greatly extends the content and the obligations of psychiatry – to the human relations of normal people, in politics, national and international, between races . . . in every form of human relationship, whether between individuals or between groups'. Twenty years ago these were visions that at times stirred up anxieties about 'psychiatry unlimited'. Today they seem to me the inescapable implications of our work. They may represent at first sight rather distant objectives, but as we proceed with the more immediate extensions that are needed in our roles as psychotherapists I believe that the action programmes the remoter

59

goals require will emerge more realistically and more urgently. I do not wish to take up this topic further at this point beyond saying that part of this programme is already in being and is now covered by the term *social psychiatry*.

Social psychiatry is, as Redlich and Freedman (1966) have put it, 'the study of the impact of the social environment on the aetiology and treatment of abnormal behaviour . . .'. Redlich adds that within this general notion there are several segmental endeavours and interests the boundaries between which are fuzzy. Social psychiatry cannot be sharply delineated from epidemiology, administrative psychiatry, preventive psychiatry, and so forth.

Community psychiatry, as Viola Bernard (1964) has stated, ' . . . is often used interchangeably with social psychiatry but is usefully distinguished from it despite the many areas of overlap between the two. It is best used to signify the applied practice at the community level, and, I believe, especially the programmes for maximizing the resources of the community towards providing direct *services* for those in need.'

In selecting these terms to give us a preliminary vocabulary, I must emphasize how tentative they are; in such a complex and comprehensive field of study as human interaction, they cannot be otherwise. What we can say is that underlying the overall ferment of activity that they represent is an increased understanding of the person not as an isolated individual, but as a being whose functioning must be viewed against the networks of social interaction in which he grows and lives. This 'third revolution in psychiatry' is a logical development from that second one that began when Freud showed that the psychological disorders of the adult could be correlated with failures in his social development. These views had a profound impact on the social sciences, which in turn began to bring new knowledge of how social forces affect behaviour. The result has been that the study of the psychological disorders now emphasizes what is happening in the family, the work situation, and the community. Correspondingly, the task of creating adequate therapeutic and preventive measures in a community has to be conceived and planned comprehensively from a wide background of knowledge and with the expertise of many disciplines.

In this collaborative endeavour, the psychotherapeutic clinic must play a fundamental role and my observations on this role spring from experience at the Tavistock Clinic over the last two decades. But in what follows I shall not when using the term 'psychotherapeutic clinic' necessarily mean a separate institution, but generally the psychotherapy component in a comprehensive psychiatric service.

TASK I. PROVIDING PSYCHOTHERAPEUTIC FACILITIES FOR THE COMMUNITY

First I should like to consider the implications of the psychotherapeutic needs in the community for the psychotherapist working in community clinics such as our Health Service units.

To appraise the task of providing adequate therapeutic facilities, it is useful to set out some of the essential features of the psychological disorders – even though these are so familiar to all of us.

(a) By 'disorder' is meant a condition in the individual in which his functioning is felt by him, or by others, to be impaired in a way that needs the help of a specially skilled person to remedy it. In any comprehensive psychiatric service, many different therapeutic methods will be valued. However much drugs or physical methods reduce feelings of stress, the need for psychotherapeutic help remains in practically all cases. By psychotherapy I mean the personal relationship with a professional person in which those in distress can share and explore the nature of their troubles, and possibly change some of the determinants, through experiencing unrecognized forces in themselves.

(b) The incidence of psychological disorders is widespread and demands for help are likely to increase as awareness of their manifestations grows. This high incidence of itself precludes sufficient help being offered in specialist centres.

(c) The psychological disorders comprise a wide range of severity and complexity both in their underlying causes and treatment. Various 'levels' of skill can therefore be appropriate in providing help. The highest level of skill is ordinarily available in the psychotherapeutic clinic where the specially trained psychotherapist is based. Less specialized psychological help is given in many other professional roles.

(d) Breakdown is governed by an interplay of both individual and social factors and it is therefore particularly liable to occur at 'crises' or points of change in the 'life space'. Help must be available at these times because the opening up of inadequate defensive patterns can often permit new growth processes to take place, both in the individual and the family.

(e) The nature of much disorder manifests itself indirectly. Help is frequently sought on the wrong basis and those offering help may collude in the avoidance of the important issues.

(f) Many pathogenic social situations are unrecognized or denied, or are left to look after themselves. For instance, one member of the family in the disturbed role hides the trouble elsewhere. Again, tensions in one section of the work organization, e.g. in senior management, may be covered up as the cause of stress elsewhere; or massive movements of the population may be treated chiefly as an economic problem with a consequent neglect of the social and psychological implications.

(g) Even when dysfunction is recognized, resistance to change, both in the individual and in social groups or organizations, is the rule and presents a specific problem requiring special procedures.

Such considerations, and they are by no means exhaustive, force us inescapably to certain conclusions about how the task of providing more therapeutic facilities must be tackled.

1. As stated, it is obvious that specially trained psychotherapists in clinics cannot deal with the situation by adhering to their original role, in which they confine themselves to work with individual patients. There must be *a large number of readily available sources of help* throughout the community. The specialist psychotherapeutic clinic is not, and cannot be, the only source of skilled help.

2. *These sources must comprise a range of different settings and roles.* Because psychological disorder is commonly manifested in a specific section of the individual's life, help is sought from various sources according to the nature of the trouble. For instance, a manifestation of tension may be taken to the family doctor, a delinquent child to the probation officer, or a psychosexual or marital problem may be presented at a family planning clinic.

Many different professions and agencies are already involved in helping individuals and families and their great advantage is that they are the most acceptable sources for those in trouble especially at times of crisis. The important issue here is the extent to which these groups can increase their contribution in quality and quantity.

3. *More skilled contribution* from the various professional groups, and especially as their work concentrates on the family and its social setting, *entails progressively more co-operation amongst them and between them and the specialist centres.* One or more workers will often be involved at one time, and more so over a period, with one family. Initial therapeutic work may lead to the uncovering of more serious problems with the need to get help from the specialist centre. This help may take the form of consultation between the psychotherapist and the field workers whereby the latter are enabled to handle the problems themselves; or it may mean that the treatment is taken over by the centre. It is therefore important that the process through which people get help should be felt as preserving a continuity. The specialist centre must not be perceived in the community as doing something quite different in character from other agencies.

Optimal collaboration and flexibility in the use of resources must be achieved and this can be done only by fulfilling certain conditions

(i) All the professional sources of help must *share the framework* on which their therapeutic work is based. All, including the specialist centre, have therefore to formulate and communicate their working hypotheses in terms of the data of human relationships. No single theoretical system needs to be adopted, but all must know the significant phenomena that have to be considered and what is involved in treating them. Moreover, the vocabulary of everyday life is normally adequate for this purpose.

(ii) *A permanent process of consultative relationships* between all sections and the specialist centre must be maintained. Psychotherapeutic relationships, at whatever level of skill, impose uncertainties and stresses on all professional personnel who get involved with the strong emotional pressures of others. Increasing their skills is a constant aim of all, but unlike the acquisition of instrumental skills, learning in this field, like the psychotherapeutic work itself, needs ongoing personal relationships of trust within a group of colleagues and between them and those on whom they rely for consultation.

(iii) *An active commitment to a permanent system of collaborative endeavour* must therefore come from the centres of highest skill. The growth of these consultant relationships with allied professional groups has to proceed voluntarily in the first instance. The situation will soon demand, however, more organization of resources both to get the largest amount of help from those available and also to conserve the scarce specialist resources. I believe that, as Rachel Levine (1966) has suggested, bodies having the function of local Mental Health Councils will have to be formed to get the most effective use of all professional personnel in any one area.

4. The fact that the kind of help given by the various professional groups for the psychological disorders has a common factor of dealing with conflicts in human relationships, and that this work begins to be perceived as closely connected with what goes on in the specialist psychological clinics, is of vital importance in getting the community to be more accepting of the nature and results of human conflicts and of the resources that people have for doing something constructive about them.

All those in familiar, respected, and trusted roles must be involved in a manifestly joint endeavour with the treatment of psychological disorders. Otherwise they are colluding in, and are seen to be colluding in, the defences by which our society splits off, and denies the recognition of, what is happening psychologically to its own members.

Resistances to the explicit awareness of the psychological nature of so much ill health and stress are a notorious obstacle to the development of the very services the community needs. Campaigns to popularize mental health knowledge are apt to have only limited success in attaining their objectives as the Cummings (1957) have demonstrated. The helping professions have a crucial role in overcoming these traditional attitudes by bringing their work into a more obvious relationship with each other and with what the specialist psychotherapeutic services are about.

The initiation of important changes is frequently stimulated when *all the necessary facts* are communicated unequivocally to those concerned. Defences against confrontation by the nature and scale of the psychological disorders are much less likely to be maintained when a growing body of respected members of the community share in both the assembling of the data for all to see and in a determination to tackle the real problems constructively and realistically within the community.

TASK 2. WHAT CAN BE DONE AMONG THE ALLIED PROFESSIONAL GROUPS?

From what has been outlined, a key role of the specialist centre is the training of allied professional personnel. Assisting these groups to increase their *knowledge* of mental ill health has long been a widespread activity of psychiatrists. To teach an appropriate psychotherapeutic *skill*, however, has not been a major effort, partly because effective, practicable methods have not been available and partly because such an expansion of skills has raised many issues of professional policy. In the early stages of psychoanalytic psychotherapy there was great reluctance on the part of its practitioners to have their knowledge applied in any 'diluted form', a concern that was justifiable as the traditional caution of any professional group.

The development of therapeutic or mental health teams inside the child guidance clinics has shown that psychotherapeutic skills can be shared when a setting is found in which the interests of all parties can be protected. There are, however, important differences when the various professional groups are in independent roles in other settings, in particular, the critical issues of responsibility and the kind of skill to be taught. It has been our view, and this is now widely accepted, that professional responsibility for what he undertakes must rest with the professional worker, not only because it is quite impracticable for the psychiatrist to take it, but because responsible skills can be acquired only when responsibility is taken. Moreover, the specialist psychotherapist in the clinic is not in a position to know the ways in which psychotherapeutic skill can best be used in the various settings of other professional groups. To take the specialist model for psychotherapy, especially the orthodox analytic psychotherapeutic one, would be manifestly unsuitable. For instance, most of the professional relationships of the family doctor introduce the complications of close physical and social contacts with the patient and his family. Again, the family social worker has usually to deal with more than one member of the family, and has often to give practical help in a variety of ways.

We have found the training methods developed and fully described by Michael Balint (1957) to be eminently practical ones for allied professional groups, and they have been used by us extensively for the last fifteen years. As Michael Balint has written, 'the skill to be acquired is not theoretical knowledge, but a personal skill and this entails a limited, though considerable, change in the personality'.

In this method, the professional workers meet weekly in groups of ten to twelve over a period of about two years for discussion of their ongoing attempts to give help. The sessions are not allowed to become therapeutic meetings, but making the group aware at times of how it reacts in tackling a member's account forms an essential part of the procedure. Understanding of how conflicting needs are expressed in human relationships thus goes hand in hand with the personal experience of experimenting with the relationships the members make with their own clients. Discussion of situations in which they have felt blocked brings for all members opportunities to scrutinize their own attitudes, and to modify these. To go back to further sessions with their clients and to bring the consequences for subsequent discussion maintains a dynamic learning process that combines new insights and skills with what is appropriate to the setting in which they are used.

A two-year period appears to be adequate for most members to work through the excitements of new powers, the 'depression' of coming up against their limitations, and then to reach a stage at which they can feel at ease with themselves in the new problems they tackle. To have benefited repeatedly from the inevitable self-revelation that is entailed in seeking advice on the handling of cases creates both a readiness to continue using consultative help and a model for their own work.

Specialist psychotherapists in the clinic who take on this kind of commitment to the professional groups in its area should have expertise in a range of psychotherapeutic work with individuals and families and in group dynamics. Our experience has shown that considerable skill can be acquired by all professional groups in the mental health field when they are given the kind of training outlined and are provided with the right setting. This latter is one in which skills can be practised with free access to the staff of the specialist clinic whom they have come to trust. The boundaries which a professional worker will set with regard to the complexity of the problems he will treat will expand with experience. The availability of regular consultation services enables him to advance under conditions of safety for all parties.

We have also found that a common framework for understanding the psychological problems of individuals and families has in fact been of great value in facilitating the sharing of cases and families and accepting the work of members of other groups. Rivalries and tensions between members of different professional groups tend to be magnified when the nature of the skills that each group practises is not known to the other, or is of such a personal and intuitive kind that members of one group cannot communicate either within their own groups or with colleagues in other groups.

Consulting services of this kind soon acquire a multiplier effect. Senior caseworkers, both in the clinic and in other agencies, with good experience and training can themselves act as group leaders for their less experienced colleagues. With groups for group leaders, the clinic staff can help in improving training skills as well as keeping in close touch with a widening range of skill training.

As a result of such steps, the Tavistock Clinic has had a programme in which about 500 professional personnel have been attending weekly meetings during each of the last few years. These groups have included family doctors, specialist doctors working in other services such as with children or in family planning clinics, health visitors, social and family caseworkers of all kinds. Groups were also drawn from the staffs of schools, approved schools, and correctional institutions, and from the clergy and others.

For this whole endeavour, the staff time required has been the equivalent of about two whole-time psychiatrists and three whole-time senior caseworkers.

Developments Associated with Increasing Psychotherapeutic Skills in the Allied Professions

More intensive psychological work by the professional workers in the community carries immediate implications for the psychotherapist with regard to the conditions and administrative arrangements for the work. The size of case loads has to be reduced, and arrangements for regular consultative sessions within their own groups and with specialists have to be 'built into' the working conditions and not left as a spare-time 'luxury'. More comprehensive case work also brings, as a rule, the need for flexibility in the type of case accepted, because people learn of its value and recommend the case worker, or the agency, to their friends.

When professional agencies adopt training programmes as described, the staff of the clinic may have to play a part in ensuring that the implications are fully examined by all those affected. New skills for the field workers often change the relationships between them and their seniors, and between all the professional staffs of an agency and its administrative authorities. As a rule it is essential for the clinic staff to participate actively in discussions of these matters with the senior administrators of the services concerned.

Questions may arise whether or not the right professional roles are available. Thus, while the role of the family doctor has tended to get lost with the rapid development of medical technology, all experience confirms his uniquely important role because of his involvement with the family at times of most stress. It has been an impressive experience to my colleagues and myself to see how many of our family doctors want to acquire psychological understanding and skill in handling psychological and family problems. The acquisition of many powerful therapeutic measures for the common illnesses has fortunately appeared to increase rather than decrease this interest. With new skills for helping emotional troubles, the general practitioner role may recover some of its appeal, for these skills can bring deep satisfaction from his greater contribution as a family caretaker.

Caretaking functions through ongoing relationships with the family, whether or not a particular member is seeking help, have assumed much more importance today with the detachment of so many families from their usual connexions. The clergy, for example, have special opportunities of this kind, e.g. in times of grief and mourning, and at marriage. With the necessary training their role enables them to offer guidance and help that might otherwise not be given.

Most important in this connexion are those services which

have prolonged contact with the individual, such as education. The growth of counselling functions within the schools and universities creates the same needs for ongoing training and close collaboration with the clinic.

The spread of facilities within the community may also expose a need for new types of service either within existing agencies or by creating new units. The Family Discussion Bureau was developed as a new type of agency after a group of social workers asked our clinic to train them to deal with the recurrent marital problems they encountered in an agency that offered an advice service to families. In the first stages the social workers had to work together with the psychiatrists to define some of the problems, to work out an adequate conceptual formulation of their nature, and then to develop methods of skill training, along with the kind of conditions required. After a few years there emerged a case work agency that embodied a workable pattern for a service for marital problems, an essential feature being regular weekly discussions with their psychiatrists.

This model attracted considerable attention and the Bureau soon had to devote a large share of its effort to training staff in other social work agencies. It showed that trained social workers, by creating a group that provided its members with support in the inevitable stresses and strains imposed by intensive case work, could acquire a very useful level of skill in handling the quite complicated marital interactions that were often presented.

As I mentioned earlier, I believe that the furthering of developments will require the professional services in an area to be co-ordinated by some kind of local Mental Health Council. The psychotherapist should play a key role in such a body. In doing so he should demonstrate by his own mode of participation in the common endeavour how constructive solutions to problems may be reached. Sensitive recognition of the interpersonal and intergroup tensions that are inevitably exposed at times, and a genuine mutuality in pooling knowledge and skills, must be his regular contribution.

Implications of these Developments for Therapeutic Work in the Clinic

I have referred to extensions to the psychotherapist's role in work outside the clinic. When the clinic becomes a focal point in the services to the community, the psychotherapist's own work has to be related to these developments. Demands for psychotherapy increase as services are created outside, not only because agencies refer patients but also as a result of the greater awareness that 'something can be done' for many disorders. Intensive individual psychotherapy has to be undertaken with a proportion of cases because this technique is one of our most important sources of understanding. However, patients for this work should be chosen in some measure so that they represent classes of problems in the community. Clinics might, for instance, plan to work on certain problems of local importance rather than for each member to adhere entirely to the usual rather random range of work. Analytical group therapy can become a major psychotherapeutic method with many assets. The experience it provides of neurotic interaction in relationships is invaluable in handling similar behaviour in disturbed marriages and in the family. Apart from its contribution to therapy it serves as an invaluable training component in group dynamics, so necessary in conducting training groups.

The choice of the family as the focus of therapy with children and adolescents is now taken as the rule. In recent years this approach for patients who are being returned from hospital to their families, even after the more serious psychotic illnesses, has been shown to be an important advance. We have found, too, that for a considerable proportion of adult psychoneurotic patients presenting with common symptoms and character problems, apparently 'individual' in nature, it is useful to examine the marital situation. With many patients the intolerable parts of themselves are collusively projected into the partner so that they are never brought into treatment. To deal with the contribution of both to what is happening can frequently end a source of resistance that makes work with the individual difficult, and at the same time mobilize the therapeutic resources of both.

This new emphasis with all patients on family interactions is a major advance in psychotherapeutic work. It becomes essential when the psychotherapist is engaged in consultative services with groups whose main work is with families. Unless its staff are keeping ahead in work that has much in common with that of the allied professional services, the clinic cannot provide the expertise that these groups need. Within the clinic, the mental health team comprising different professional skills becomes of paramount importance in this respect, with its demonstration of how the therapeutic skills of all members can be maintained at a high level.

Work with families also highlights the need for the consultant psychotherapist to understand intergroup as well as intragroup dynamics, for the family group functions in a network of inter-group relations. When he works with larger social organizations, e.g. with staffs of residential institutions, knowledge of intergroup dynamics is indispensable.

Compared with his traditional role, the specialist psycho-therapist in the community clinic has therefore to acquire a much broader experience within the clinic of different therapeutic endeavours. He has also to learn much more of how the com-munity served by the clinic functions. It may be added that in our experience this broader experience, far from detracting from his basic skills, tends to give him a sharpened appreciation of how best to use these.

TASK 3. CREATING THE CONDITIONS FOR THE OPTIMAL
DEVELOPMENT AND FUNCTIONING OF THE PER-
SONALITY: PREVENTION

Access to many powerful forces in the personality is only to be obtained when the person is in the security of a therapeutic relationship. Accordingly, the role of the psychotherapeutic clinic in providing a laboratory for the study of the development of the individual personality, and hence for knowledge on which primary preventive measures could be based, needs no further comment here.

That a much wider relationship must be developed by the clinic to the problems of aetiology and hence of prevention, and the development of positive mental health measures, becomes clearer the more the effects of social factors on the functioning of the person are studied.

To illustrate this theme I shall take some recent findings on work stress and work satisfaction. Investigating the high in-cidence of stress manifested in certain groups of miners, Trist and his colleagues (Trist, 1963) showed that a new technology in the mines had broken up the traditional working groups and replaced them by work roles and groups based primarily on the

machines. After prolonged working through of the various implications of change, a new social organization was then designed
that retrieved the old self-regulating patterns for small work
groups and yet at the same time was appropriate for the demands
of the machines. The result was a marked fall in sickness and
absenteeism rates, a recovery of work satisfaction and a rise in
productivity. Further work has emphasized this need to view the
work group as a *socio-technical system*, to use Trist's term, i.e. as
a system in which the social and personal needs of the worker
must be satisfied by a work setting that simultaneously meets the
technological requirements. Responsible participation in social
tasks appears to exert a major influence on the feelings of security
and competence in the individual.

Again, Menzies's (1960) investigation of the high wastage rate
in training nurses suggests that the pattern of the nurse's work
that has developed in recent years represents a social system
evolved to act as a powerful defence against the emergence of
feelings that are felt to be uncontrollable. In this particular case
the defence not only denied the feelings involved, the emotions
inevitably associated with the 'nursing relationship', but the
system also deprived the nurse of the necessary reassurance that
the work could have given in response to these feelings. In other
words, the system failed to deal with the primary anxiety aroused
and created a secondary anxiety from frustration and the inhibition
of creative development.

This kind of study, and an enormous mass of other findings,
raise many aspects of the relation between psychotherapy and
the social sciences.

Affinities between the clinic and the social sciences have become
clearer as group methods have been used by the psychotherapists.
It is not only small groups, however, that can be described as
microsociology. Detailed psychotherapeutic work shows that the
study of the person can also be categorized in this way. The personality carries within it dynamically structured object-relations
that mediate a range of 'social' relationships with figures belong-
ing to the inner world; the patterns of relationship with people
in the outer world closely resemble these inner structures. These
theories in turn have led to several creative lines of thought on
the functioning of small groups in regard to the deeper forces
influencing relations both between members and between mem-

bers and the leader. It is highly significant that the most profound contributions to our understanding of small groups have come from psychoanalysts. Leading sociologists, e.g. Talcott Parsons and Bales (1955), have interestingly enough reached similar conclusions.

Personality theory must be extended from the sphere of intrapsychic dynamics if we are to account for the range and quality of the needs to belong in various groups, to achieve, and to define and maintain a satisfying identity and self-feeling in co-operative relations with others in significant activities. Clinical work suggests that the integrity of the central self is usually achieved at the expense of splitting off parts of the personality that embody repressed needs for relationship. In spite of the familiar defence mechanisms, many of these needs remain as unconscious compulsions to recreate relationships in which they can be satisfied. The objects for these relationships are often selected from the groups in which people live or work. Such relationships may possibly underlie the 'social atom' that Moreno (1956) has found to characterize group relatedness. Again, the need to exert some mastery over these inner relationships may be connected with the kind of satisfaction many people require in work, e.g. the feeling of being a responsible member of a self-regulating group. As automation progresses, new means of satisfying social needs will have to be evolved. To all these problems, the psychotherapeutic clinic has a unique contribution to make. But it does mean that the psychotherapist has to pay much more attention to the psychodynamic contribution of the social *milieu* to the functioning of the individual.

In our modern world, change has to become a normal and positive experience in many areas of living. Social scientists and administrators on the whole have been much more able to diagnose what has to be changed than to manage a successful change process. If we remind ourselves that, as Jaques and others have described, the characteristics of many social systems have been evolved in substantial measure to deal with the threatening tensions within them, then we will be prepared for the consequences of trying to change it. All psychotherapists are familiar with the anxieties aroused within the individual when he begins to alter his defence systems. It is inevitable that such alterations within the defensive patterns of a social system will also release anxiety and a degree of 'acting-out'. Social systems can create special difficulties during the change process; but individuals within it can also give each other considerable positive support during change.

New satisfactions have to be experienced and accepted before old ways can be given up, and during this process the role of a therapeutic person or group of persons has a close parallel with the role occupied by the therapist for the individual or the family. Our experience has therefore been that the social scientist who wishes to be involved in change processes has to acquire, in addition to his knowledge, a skill that enables him to maintain a professional relationship while these change processes with their inevitable anxieties and 'acting-out' are being initiated and worked through. Such skills naturally have to be evolved with special experience, but the psychotherapeutic relationship, especially in analytic group therapy, can provide a valuable basic model. Some social scientists may seek personal analysis as a foundation, but, where this is not adopted, experience, even as observers of therapeutic groups over a long period, is extremely useful as a foundation for professional skills.

Administrators, and others occupying key managerial roles, have also to be offered skill training in human relations.

The whole conceptual basis for research and development into the tasks of improving the social environment has fundamental problems that are common to the psychotherapist and the social scientist. Close collaboration between them must therefore be a part of the activities of the psychological clinic. The psychotherapeutic clinic has a unique role as a control mechanism picking up critical data on damage being done within the current social processes. Use cannot be made of this role, however, unless the clinic is integrated with a wider group of institutions in the community, and especially those that can value its findings and on this basis initiate changes. In other words, while a comprehensive mental health endeavour may undo some of the rejection by society of its psychological disorders, there is a danger that new services may develop merely 'within' the community yet still relatively isolated from it, instead of getting into the integrated relationship with key institutions that is required.

The location of the clinic within its social space therefore assumes a new importance. It would seem that it has to become one component in a constellation of units – which together share the task of attaining a better society. The psychotherapist is still apt to be regarded as a mystery man, and one of his obligations is to undo some of this attribution by fostering these interrelationships. In these new roles, however, his increased experience and knowledge merely add to the basic pattern of his relationships with others. That is to say, he does not tell others what to do, but by helping them to expose the unrecognized forces in social relationships he shares with them a fully collaborative task.

SUMMARY

Expanding community mental health services and working towards better community mental health entail new roles for the psychotherapeutic clinic. Its staff have to initiate and maintain a large-scale training programme whereby the psychotherapeutic skill of all the helping professions can be raised. The clinic has then to remain a focal point in maintaining an increasing level of competence throughout this system. Inside the clinic, psychotherapeutic practice, besides preserving the traditional role of providing long-term individual treatment for some, must comprise work that closely parallels much of the work in the community. High expertise must be maintained in the treatment of the family, in group therapy, and in group dynamics. Lastly, because of its role in picking up the breakdowns from the current social processes, it occupies a unique position to act as a servo-mechanism, which must be integrated with key institutions and other disciplines, for evolving comprehensive knowledge through which the community can take in hand more effectively the formulation of its values and the shaping of its own destiny around them.

REFERENCES

BALINT, M. (1957). *The doctor, his patient, and the illness.* London: Pitman Medical Publishing Co.

BELLAK, L. (ed.) (1964). *Handbook of community psychiatry and community mental health.* New York: Grune and Stratton.

BERNARD, V. (1964). In L. Bellak (ed.) *supra.*

CUMMING, J., & E. (1957) *Closed ranks.* Cambridge, Mass.: Harvard University Press.

GREGG, A. (1944). *American Journal of Psychiatry.*

LEVINE, R. (1966). *American Journal of Psychiatry.*

MENZIES, I. E. P. (1960). Case-study in the functioning of social systems as a defence against anxiety: a report of a study on the nursing service of a general hospital. *Hum. Relat.* **13,** 95–121.

MORENO, J. L. (1956). *Sociometry and the science of man.* New York: Beacon House.

PARSONS, TALCOTT, & BALES, R. F. (1955). *Family, socialization and interaction process.* London: Routledge and Kegan Paul.

REDLICH, F. C. & FREEDMAN, D. X. (1966). *The theory and practice of psychiatry.* New York: Basic Books.

TRIST, E. L. *et al.* (1963). *Organizational choice.* London: Tavistock Publications.

6 The Changing Role of the Social Worker

BARBARA BUTLER

The image of the social worker has changed: 'she' is now a third as likely to be a 'he', and far more likely to have with-it gear than a hat and flat shoes, and is as likely to be young as middle-aged.

Social workers come from a variety of training backgrounds too, as well as being varied creatures; and the patterns of training that produce them are changing all the time. In 1967 there were about twelve thousand social workers (excluding residential staff) employed in the statutory services, and about three thousand more should by now (1970) have completed their training (Dept. of Health and Social Security, 1968, appendices L and M). After allowances are made for 'loss through marriage' and other causes, and for the appointment of untrained personnel, just about one-third altogether have had trainings recognized by the Home Office Central Training Council in Child Care or the Probation Training Committee, by the Ministry of Health, by the Council for Training in Social Work, or by certain of the professional organizations. The range is from two years of specialized theory and practice in the social studies and human relationships – often taken by graduates in related humanities, or by people already practising social work – to, at the farther extreme, a three months' period of theoretical study within the frame of several months of supervised social work; or even, earlier, to a series of day-release and weekend courses within a similar framework.

This leaves several thousand workers with no formal training apart from any in-service training that may be given. There was in 1966 a projected need by 1970 of about one-third of the total again; trained or, presumably, untrained. Great efforts are being made to provide courses adequate in both quality and quantity

77

to meet this need; but many of the people sought are of the same kind as teachers, doctors, lawyers, and other professionals in whom intelligence and integrity are required and for whom society's need is great.

In addition to the changes in kind and demand, social workers are also having to establish their role in a context of fundamental changes within the administrative structures in which they function. The most extensive of these changes are the result of the Local Authority Personal Services Act (1970); this requires the reorganization of departments within the pattern of wider administrative reforms in local government and in the national health services. Earlier examples are the changes consequent upon the London local authorities' reorganization; the readjustment of services following the 1959 Mental Health Act and the 1963 and 1969 Children and Young Persons Acts are yet others that combined to create an environment where expectations were confused – and we all know what happens to people when several contradictory expectations are imposed on them!

In addition to such external complications there are the social workers' own confusions about themselves, only partially resolved during the formation in 1970 of the British Association of Social Workers. This Association is the outcome of a thirty-year-long history of attempts to bring together the various branches of social work; in 1964 the eight major groups created the Standing Conference of Organizations of Social Work, and from the labours of this Standing Conference has emerged the British Association with its membership of over eleven thousand social workers. This is after all appropriate. There are in social work at its best the proper attributes of a profession; systematic knowledge, valued technical skill, and trained capacity to work in the service of others. The Government's White Paper concerned with the rearrangement of Scottish personal social services following the Kilbrandon Report (Scottish Home and Health Dept., 1964) recognized this specifically, 'social workers are increasingly taking the view – and this is being reflected in training arrangements – that social work is a single profession within which specialities should be subordinate to the profession as a whole, in much the same way as medical specialities are subordinate to the profession of medicine' (Scottish Home and Health Dept., 1966).

That Committee took this view so seriously that they suggested placing Probation Officers along with Child Care Officers within the family welfare services of the local authorities; they also recommended that the proposed Directors of Social Work should be chief officers. These recommendations were all implemented in the radical Social Work (Scotland) Act 1969. There is in fact little misunderstanding at central government level of the overall role that social workers should be expected to adopt. The various reports, such as the Macintosh (Macintosh, 1951), Kilbrandon (*op. cit.*), Younghusband (Ministry of Health, 1959), Ingleby (Home Office, 1960), and Morison (Home Office, 1962), all contain references and descriptions of social work that even those of us responsible for training social workers can recognize. What is not understood is that if social work practice of the kind and availability recognized as desirable is to be provided, then re-organization of public funds is necessary. There is a need for redeployment of financial resources in two main areas: to ensure that the training of social workers and the departments they work in are adequately funded, tasks for the new Councils under the Seebohm Act; and, far more importantly, to ensure that real shifts are made to meet the shamefully continuing needs of socially deprived areas. At present a major part of the personal social services' time, energy, and other resources are devoted to attempts to relieve stress situations almost entirely due to economic conditions, situations that would send any of us dotty overnight. This is particularly true of the great abnormal industrial connurbations among which London is the greatest. It is an old adage that a people gets the government it deserves. It is equally true that governments are faced with the problems people create through their curiously distorted value systems. We now are faced with a wide range of damaged people and disordered relationships rooted in the last quarter century and before. Even if, for instance, the reforms suggested by the Child Poverty Action Group (1966) are put into practice and Family Allowances are raised, even if educational systems are improved, community living fostered, housing made adequate, and the national income increased through demonstrable economic productivity, there is still left with us the fundamental problem of all those many individuals in disordered relationships, few of them 'well enough' for us to feel at all happy about them and their lack of abundance of life. Nations, as well as individuals, have to make their choice about whether to be on the side of life or death. Even though we are probably better off than in the darkest days of the Industrial Revolution and Chadwick's 'Insanitary Conditions', nevertheless, a question *is* raised here for social workers. They are in daily contact with people suffering from considerable environmental stresses; what reformative action can and should they take? I should like to return to this point later, and to continue now with the role of the social workers as seen by themselves.

Rogers and Dixon (1960) in their 'Portrait of Social Work' in the north of England, and Jeffreys (1965) in her study in the south, all convey a picture of confused allocation of roles and functions between different local authority service agencies; and also between them and the hospital and court services. The further point that comes across, and is constantly experienced in practice, is that there is generally not enough trust or understanding of each other's specialist function between different kinds of differently trained social workers, with a consequent lowering of service to the consumers. This is not a characteristic of social work only. In many places concerted attempts are being made in small groups and larger conferences to improve the nature of this trust and understanding by sharing common tasks and problems. A model of such experience has been offered, for instance, by the national biennial study conferences organized by the Association of Social Workers and subsequently published (Association of Social Workers, 1963, 1965, 1967, 1969). At a more local level, the case conference system enables some of the barriers of specialization to be lessened, giving occasions for all workers from different agencies who are concerned with particular families to meet to produce the most constructive and relevant treatment plan. Surely the families too ought sometimes to be represented at such case conferences?

So far I have been mainly discussing social workers in general and the problems caused by varied trainings, lack of trainings, and changing expectations and environments, with a passing reference to the consequent difficulties between social workers themselves and between them and other related professions.

Now I want to narrow my discussion to that proportion of social workers who can be said to be fully trained, whatever setting they practice in. By 'fully trained' I mean that they have spent at least fifteen months after graduation, or more probably at least two years, preparing themselves to do their specialist jobs; and that for a fair part of this time they have learned from responsible practice under regular close supervision. These are people who have had the opportunity to acquire the real expertise of a profession, and who can speak with the proper authority of the specialist about human relationships in society. The group most familiar to many readers will probably be psychiatric social workers; and though I shall be examining in particular their changing role, I should like to make it clear that in considering the functioning of the mental health team, I would expect as much weight to be given to the contribution of any other fully trained social worker as to that of the psychiatric social worker. As far back as 1956, the London and South East branch of the Association of Psychiatric Social Workers commented on the generic training course started at the London School of Economics in 1954 thus,

'We think that all branches of social casework nowadays require the kind of skill and training hitherto only afforded to psychiatric social workers, and the programme of the first generic course as it has been described to us encourages us to think that these needs may now be to some extent met . . . We do not see an essential difference between the theoretical concepts of social casework and psychiatric social work.'

Social casework training has gone on apace since then; and while standards between training institutions vary, as do those of teaching hospitals, nevertheless the general standard is probably adequate. Student psychiatric social workers themselves now often, and rightly in my view, form one branch among several on the various generic courses. This demonstrates the likemindedness of the basic professional skills and knowledge needed; and psychiatry is included as a common course for all students whether they become child care officers, probation officers, psychiatric social workers, family caseworkers, or medical social workers.

Having acknowledged these similarities, I am nevertheless going to discuss particularly that distinct and specific group of social workers called psychiatric social workers. For one thing, this has been the most self-consciously articulate group; and for another, I suspect that they offer a model for what may happen generally in the personal social services to all social workers whose professional qualifications are recognized.

As Timms (1964) has described in his history of the Association of Psychiatric Social Workers, definition of function has occupied an important place in their writings. My own impression, reading through nearly twenty years of journals, is of a persistent attempt by generous-minded, well-educated spokesmen to broaden the minds of their less flexible colleagues. The pattern of changing roles put on psychiatric social workers by their training experiences, by the expectations of their medical colleagues, and by the demands of the community through changing legislation are faithfully reflected. There is constant reiteration in the early years of the fact that they are trained to work in a team, at first the main stated task being to provide social histories for the doctors, then to do treatment with parents, and even sometimes to venture to treat children too. In hospital teams the move has been towards increasing links with employers and other social agencies, towards more work with relatives and treatment through groups. Following the 1959 Mental Health Act, there is increasing discussion of the role the psychiatric social worker must take as consultant to less knowledgeable social workers of all kinds, as the link between the hospital and the rest of the world (demonstrated by the creation of joint-user appointments) and as the specialist social worker helping the more disordered patients still functioning outside hospital. In the cases presented as examples of ways of working, the situations described read more and more as if they came from the case loads of any other professional social worker in the community; and the psychiatric social worker seems to work increasingly independently, even when based on child guidance clinics.

There is a curious reluctance to meet certain challenges, such as that of statutory duties parallel to those carried out by child care officers or probation officers. De Mesurier (1949) exposes some interesting assumptions, writing of psychiatric social workers acting as Duly Authorized Officers, when she says:

' . . . some of our profession feel that the Duly Authorized Officer's duties are as remote from psychiatric social work as are the duties of a constable on the beat . . . The power to make quick decisions, to improvise action in a crisis, to impose our will on another person, is definitely not to be acquired by studying human relationships, therapeutic approach or passive technique.'

I think that probably over the last fifteen years much of this problem of authority has been clarified and so better understood and better handled (see e.g. Hunt, 1962). It seems, too, as if there are still many psychiatric social workers (and others, such as probation officers) who could usefully remember Goldberg's views:

'We psychiatric social workers became deeply absorbed in the use of our therapeutic relationship with the individual client, while withdrawing more and more from the hurlyburly of the slums, and the overcrowded rooms (or respectable villas) of our clients; into the consulting room; viewing visiting, for instance, as an inferior form of casework in which psycho-analytic insight could not be applied' (Goldberg, 1955).

Irvine (1959) goes further towards indicating the variety of helping ways open to social workers, would they only use them, when she says of two contributors to the Association's journal:

' . . . both these authors are concerned with the rediscovery and rehabilitation of matters which for some time have been neglected and undervalued on account of an interest in intro-spective techniques and the deeper level of transference . . . of value to neurotic clients; . . . but for many of those presenting marked degrees of immaturity, psychopathy or borderline psychotic conditions, deeds speak louder than words, and the worker must play an active role if his reality is to reach the client through the fog of discouraging experience and the mirages of alarming phantasy. But these methods lack pres-tige . . .'

Her later paper 'What is Advanced Casework?' argues very persuasively that real skill lies in having a wide range of helping techniques available and in responding with them appropriately to the wide range of needs presented by people in distress (Irvine, 1962).

This shift towards eclecticism in practice is slowly being accepted.

It can be seen too in the work of other members of the mental health team. Mr Phillipson's description (see Chapter 7) of the wider range of aims and techniques open to clinical psychologists is one example; and Dr Sutherland's paper included in this volume also contains in it indications of the breadth and range of techniques available to psychiatrists and other mental health specialists in their work to improve the community situation. The question is how far the training of psychiatrists is moving to include content concerned with the meaning of life and feelings and relationships in society, so as to enable them to make use of such breadth of resource. The ordinary GP is particularly handicapped through his training, though perhaps Professor Titmuss's committee will change this in the future; and the work being done in Balint-type groups to increase understanding (and perhaps humility) redresses things for only a small number (Balint, 1957). A possible way of improving the balance may be for group practices to make more use of social workers, perhaps seconded to them by Local Authorities, in order to bring team skills into general medicine. However, the problem is most relevant to psychiatrists, whose trainings have not always helped to deepen their humanity or their understanding of people in community. Traditionally the psychiatrist leads the mental health team whether in clinic, hospital, or community; and his status and prestige, i.e. his salary, is proportionate, as Beedell (1957) points out. This does not necessarily mean that he has the greatest personal authority or knowledge: to quote Beedell, a clinical psychologist, on the homogeneity of the different team members (with its consequences for communication and understanding between them):

'The psychiatric social workers are most homogeneous by virtue of their personal training and personal methods of selection. Psychiatrists are because of their medical training, but less so because of their differing psychiatric training. Psychologists are even a little startling in their variety. These disciplines differ in the intensity of training for their particular job and the amount of psychological education (in an academic sense) which goes with it. The psychiatric social workers have most; the others much less.'

Freeman (1965) also comments: 'The conventional medical education gives doctors very little understanding of the role of social workers, and scarcely even a basic knowledge of who these people are and what they do.' He discusses many of the problems arising through differences of status and shows how some of them may be lessened, mainly through greater mutual understanding.

Other writers also discuss the problem of effective teamwork between the different disciplines. Lewis (1950) remarks: 'I feel that a fixed line of demarcation between the functions of the psychiatrist and the psychiatric social worker tends to be made only when co-operation between them is not based on mutual trust.' A later study of 142 American mental health agencies concluded that 'Interprofessional competition for status, combined with uncertainty about aims, lack of training standards and suitable personnel were so frequently found as to indicate only rudimentary development of inter-disciplinary teamwork psychotherapy' (Committee on Psychotherapy, 1960). It would be tempting to say this is of course true for American agencies only; but is it? Rafferty's paper 'Symptoms and Process in the Multi-disciplined Community' (1960) is surely applicable in many ways to the English scene, with its description of the defence patterns evolved to deal with demands felt to be too great; the territoriality of catchment areas; the buckpassing from agency to agency; the tendency towards specialization: these are recognizable here too. Harrington (1961), writing of her experience in the integration of child therapy and casework, indicates that in practice 'the team' as a working unit had almost ceased to exist beyond the diagnostic stage, apart from *ad hoc* meetings concerned with crises.

I am quite sure that there are innumerable examples of good productive teamwork and many descriptions have been published of fascinating work done in a variety of team situations. Nevertheless, as if I were a therapist, I must also bring out some of the negative aspects of team experience. From them it is also possible to deduce positives and facilitate fruitful development.

One of the major problems in establishing effective teamwork is that of communication. People have to *want* to communicate in order to get through the barriers of differing experience and training. Enthusiasm for a common aim is useful, but common aims get tarnished unless regularly assessed for value and appropriateness. Clear organizational processes designed to ease formal communication, together with adequate opportunities for informal communication, are necessary if any groups of people are

G

to function towards common ends (Sofer, 1961; Rice, 1965). In established settings such as hospitals and clinics, there is normally structured into the weekly pattern of events the ward or staff or clinic meeting. This is not necessarily so in Local Authority settings; but it must be made part of the organizational process if proper sharing of specialist knowledge and mutual support against the anxieties of the job are to be achieved. This applies not just to mental health departments, but to all departments and agencies to which the endless stresses of people in difficulty and distress are brought for relief.

The less opportunity provided by the agency for the sharing and containing of anxiety in mature ways, the more difficulty there will be in providing the kind of service required to help people in need. Menzies's (1961) study of the hospital is a classic description of inappropriate and not altogether effective organizational measures to cope with such anxiety.

That the traditional pattern of the hospital, and more particularly of the child guidance, team (when it is functioning reasonably well) is a powerful factor in dealing with such anxiety situations is clearly exemplified in Woodward's (1961) comments:

'I did not appreciate how safe and comfortable it was to work in a child guidance clinic team until, after 3 years of working in one, I took up a new job in a Birmingham hospital entirely on my own – that is to say, outside the psychiatric setting. One of the first shocks was to find that in contrast to the clinic where the team shared a common language and where many working friendships were acceptable to us all, I found myself among a variety of people without apparently any shared principles on which we could all base a way of working. It made me realize how much I had taken for granted in the clinic: and more important, how few of the ideas that are accepted so easily in clinic practice are not only non-existent outside, but heartily rejected.'

Such a model of good experience of working with colleagues in different disciplines is of inestimable value when social workers transfer to the open 'multitudinous compromise situations' (Thomas, 1950) of the world outside hospitals and clinics. Models of bad experience have their value too, if the workers concerned have sufficient understanding and skill to appreciate some of the factors that make them bad and can use this understanding with imagination in new situations.

For it seems to me that one of the major roles that must be played by professional social workers *is* that of the teamworker. This, in view of the increasing tendency in psychiatric social work towards independence, and towards a wide range of techniques, may seem contradictory. But in fact the trained social caseworker can draw upon a fund of specific knowledge and skill about people in social relationship greater than that almost any other worker in the mental health team can have acquired by sole virtue of his specific training. Differences of emphasis are not however necessarily differences for better or for worse in this particular area of work, where the complexities of the problems facing the community require as much skill of all kinds as can be turned to their unravelling. To spend time isolating areas of difference and maintaining rigid demarcation lines about what is to be done by which particular kind of specialist can only create ludicrous situations of the kind that some trade union members have found themselves in. Even though the trained social worker should be expected to have a special expertise in ways of working with people in relationships, in knowledge of environmental resources, and in effective sociological factors, this is not necessarily her prerogative – any more than the understanding of academic psychology or TAT tests, or of the medical consequences of drugs or operations or illnesses, is necessarily the prerogative of psychologists or doctors. In the gradual revolution from the divine right of physical medicine to the democracy of total prophylaxis, any person able to accept the responsibilities and duties of knowledge must do so to the best of his or her ability in the sphere where knowledge can be most fully made fruitful. For the trained social worker today, this is almost certainly within the community itself more than within institutions such as prisons and hospitals, which are still at times encapsulated from the 'hurly-burly'. Child care officers and family caseworkers have always had to face this; probation officers are having increasingly to move between community and capsule; psychiatric social workers certainly have accepted this, with nearly half of them now in posts held outside hospitals or clinics; and even the most encapsulated group of all, the medical social workers, are increasingly taking posts directly in community services.

In tune with this overall shift of emphasis for the responsibility for mental health into the everyday world of ordinary people travelling on tubes and in buses, more and more often with odder and odder strangers, the mental health team itself may now contain members who might not at one time have seemed appropriate. In fact we no longer find so often 'the mental health team', familiar in hospital and clinic; rather we find teams of people working together for specific aims towards the improvement of mental health, whether on behalf of one particular person, or one family, or particular groups of people (such as housing estates, or Aberfan, or specific industries). Such teams may or may not contain professional workers of the kind we usually mean; but often it will fall to one of the 'traditional' members to act as consultant or specialist participant. Because the social worker is traditionally imbued with more ordinariness and less magic than her psychologist and psychiatrist colleagues, she may have a specially important role to fulfil in this everyday world – the role of translator and interpreter in simple terms to the ordinarily muddled people who have to live and work alongside the mentally disordered and distressed, and who may have to take considerable responsibility themselves, without necessarily having the resources of knowledge and support they need.

I want now to examine five particular areas of work where the social worker's role seems to be changing. They will not be so different in some ways from the areas in which other members of the traditional team may find themselves functioning as well. But because in the eyes of many people (including some of those who as councillors or others actually employ them) the social worker's role is seen to be more humble and is less understood than that of her colleagues, the focus may be rather different. There is now for instance often the additional problem posed by the fact that while informed colleagues *know* that a professionally trained social worker can speak with authority and will accept this, less informed people will disregard their contribution, or confuse the various kinds of trained and untrained social workers, attributing knowledge or skills or ignorance inappropriately and indiscriminately so that the social work profession has to carry the blame for much that does not rightly belong to it. Many people must experience this in other fields, for instance when lawyers discount specialist medical evidence in the courts; or when lay people assume that doctors have the skill to advise and participate in all the complexities of relationships and motives involved in adoption placements.

The first area is teamwork. During their training, and often in their practice before moving into other agencies, social workers are able to learn about functioning in a team. It may be the orthodox team of clinic or hospital; or it may be in both the probation teams, that is within the court and within the office; or it may be within the team of agency consultants and supervisors such as in Family Service Units or the Family Welfare Association, or within the more hierarchical teams and groups in children's departments: but the students will have had to learn about ways of sharing responsibility and knowledge with colleagues who may well come from different professions, or none. By being able to look at what happens in such team situations, these students can be helped to create and introject a safe model, which they can take securely into their work in different settings. When it is necessary for treatment purposes to set up an *ad hoc* team of workers of varied backgrounds, for instance of priest, district nurse, Red Cross worker, home help, and social worker, they have some experience of the kinds of problem that may arise and the ways of dealing with them. Instead of being members of one or two teams, they must be able to work in many, and often to take the responsibility for creating, containing, and maintaining such teams in operation. This makes tremendous demands. It is relatively easy to learn to work with the strengths and weaknesses of a team whose membership is fairly constant. Learning to work with many different people is a far greater challenge; knowing how to help in the clarification of aims and focus of work, how to share and to ease possible tensions and relieve misunderstandings between members is much more difficult in teams where people have not necessarily grown used to working together. Because social workers are often working at ground level, so to speak, with workers also directly in touch with clients, it is particularly important for them to know how to be teammembers and quite often how to convene such teams.

The second role to comment on is that of educator. This operates at several levels; for instance, as consultant to groups outside the employing agency, or as adviser within the agency to other less experienced members of staff and to members of the public and non-social-work members of staff. There is little need to do more than refer to the work of, for instance, Gerald Caplan (1961; 1964) for a useful discussion of consultancy within the mental health field. Experience has shown its practical value; and descriptions by, among others, Irvine (1964), Mackenzie (1963), and Moffat (1955) show the application of such ideas in England. As a point of policy it is worth remembering Irvine's discussion of the use of sanction in establishing such consultancy services: she talks of the need for allowing adequate time when introducing such services into other agencies from the specialist psycho-therapeutic unit Dr Sutherland describes elsewhere in this book, and of the need to educate the top level of administration if the middle and lower levels are to derive any meaningful benefit. Increasingly social workers are being required to bring their special knowledge and skills to bear on members of the public, not as clients but as assistants. The great surges of voluntary helper schemes are often guided by social workers more or less fitted for this skilled rather ambiguous task. To quote a few examples: the prison aftercare service is using associates to help discharged prisoners, trained through such schemes as that at the Blackfriars Settlement; Camden Council of Social Service has, like many others, developed organized training schemes for voluntary workers; Oxford City Children's Department is using supervised voluntary workers in problem families: the range is endless and is in itself a move towards positive mental health in its channelling of reparative energies to purposeful ends. The role of educator of such voluntary workers on such a scale is new, and is being increasingly accepted as proper both to members of the traditional mental health team and to other professionally trained social therapists.

This is in the community at large. Mental health work is also important within agencies and organizations of all kinds, whether factories or shops or schools or hospitals or local authority departments. Woodward's (1961) comment is particularly relevant here, 'One of the purposes a caseworker can fulfil is in helping generally to humanize the hospital (*et al.*) atmosphere by giving due recognition to the existence of *feelings* (as distinct from rules, duties, expediencies, etc.).' Only people who are able, naturally or by training, to tolerate the recognition and expression of feelings can understand the frustration experienced by those in need when they are not allowed to experience their feelings because the institution has no place for them. In this respect it may well be the duty of the social worker in particular, because of her intermediary position between agency or institution and people at large, to make more of her role of candlebearer. Her 'good deed' may be to personify recognition of the importance of feelings in positive mental health processes, when she may be working in naughty worlds dark and shuttered against such acknowledgement.

Fourthly, in the social worker's situation between the agency and people served by the agency, where she is the face-to-face mediator of administrative processes and policies to her clients, she must increasingly take over the role of the 'feeder-back': the person who can transmit information back into the agency in such a way as to enable faulty administration and policy to be changed. Certainly in training social workers, this aspect of understanding and responsibility is being increasingly emphasized. Critical studies of agency function and functioning lead them to have increasingly high standards of what good organization should be like, in order to free them to do the work they are trained to do. I mentioned earlier the need for including in a personal service agency a place for regular consultation and sharing of anxieties and resources. This is only one example of the kind of reform that professional workers are seeking to bring in as standard practice. They are often up against the problem of ill-informed lay staff or committees who have authority over them and who may not see the point of 'time for thinking'. Jones and Hammond (1960) discussing 'The Boundaries of Training' have this to say:

> 'In the Local Authority setting, the goal is less clearly defined because historically the services . . . developed primarily from the concepts of the Poor Law . . . In the Local Authority team . . . there may be officials who without any true clinical training in psychiatry are responsible for the policy of the department.'

It is perhaps only as more professionally trained workers take over senior administrative posts that real movement here can be made.

The last area of changing role I wish to comment on follows on from this and also links back to the point made earlier about the reformative action that should be part of the professional person's task. Without adequate accurate information it is impossible to make plans for community health, or for anything else, except in faith. The need for good research studies of verifiable material upon which to base coherent and constructive policies is tremendous. The Research Unit at Bedford College and the Home Office Research Unit are examples of attempts to begin to meet this need. But enough is certainly not being done to tap the resources of skill and information available in the community. Social workers are increasingly being trained to understand and take part in research projects; many have stimulated and introduced research work in their departments where none existed before. Their special skills may mean that they could be used in specific research areas – where depth interviewing is called for, for instance. But their role in research seems to be often that of conscience; it is often the social workers who will press for follow-up work to be done with people whose needs have been revealed or perhaps even exacerbated by research enquiries, for instance. Their contribution as responsible members of that group of professional people most concerned with the relief and prevention of mental ill health is increasingly recognized and made use of, so that many research projects in this field are as likely to be headed by social workers as by psychiatrists or psychologists. An example of this is the 'battered baby' research project being undertaken by the NSPCC.

To sum up, the role of social workers in the mental health team is changing, alongside that of their colleagues in this and other fields, towards greater flexibility and maturity in the use of special knowledge and skills. When all comes to all, the only thing that matters, whatever knowledge and skills we may possess, is the quality of our relationships with our fellow men and women whether as colleagues, clients, administrators, or assistants. If we are good at being people we are useful members of the mental health team, whatever we label ourselves, and whatever form the team takes.

I should like to end with some words from the Earl of Feversham's presidential address to the Association of Psychiatric Social Workers in 1961:

'A few of us now realize the tremendous denial of human rights and human dignity implicit in this refusal to do everything in our power with the knowledge and affluence now available to us to restore mentally disordered people as far as possible to normal life. The whole of our thinking and of our approach to the principles of human life is expressed in our attitudes towards mental health. Mental health is not the concern only of those who are disordered, it is the concern of every individual.'

Perhaps it is the wider sharing of this concern in a constructively reformative way that is the crux of the social worker's developing role.

REFERENCES

ASSOCIATION OF PSYCHIATRIC SOCIAL WORKERS, LONDON & S. E. BRANCH (1956). *Brit. J. psychiat. soc. Work* 3, iv, 29.
ASSOCIATION OF SOCIAL WORKERS (1963). *New thinking for changing needs.*
—— (1965). *New thinking about administration.*
—— (1967). *New thinking about institutional care.*
—— (1969). *New thinking about welfare.*
BALINT, M. (1957). *The doctor, the patient and his illness.* London: Pitman Medical Publishing Co.
BEEDELL, C. (1957). *The psychopathology of interclinic conferences.* London: National Association for Mental Health.
CAPLAN, G. (1961). *An approach to community mental health.* London: Tavistock Publications; New York: Grune & Stratton.
—— (1964). *Principles of preventive psychiatry.* London: Tavistock Publications; New York: Basic Books.
CHILD POVERTY ACTION GROUP (1966). Statement. *Case Confer.* **12**, x, 331–7.
COMMITTEE ON PSYCHOTHERAPY (1960). Report: The psychotherapeutic function of the orthopsychiatric team. *Amer. J. Orthopsychiat.* **30**, i, 49–79.
DE MESURIER (1949). The duly authorised officer. *Brit. J. psychiat. soc. Work* **1**, ii, 45–8.
DEPARTMENT OF HEALTH AND SOCIAL SECURITY (1968). *Report: Local authority and allied personal social services* (Seebohm Report). London: HMSO.

FEVERSHAM, EARL OF (1961). The changing pattern of the mental health services. *Brit. J. psychiat. soc. Work* **6**, i, 52–5.

FREEMAN, H. (ed.) (1965). *Symposium on psychiatric hospital care, London, 1964: Psychiatric hospital care.* London; Baillière, Tindall & Cassell.

GOLDBERG, E. M. (1955). Some developments in professional collaboration and research in the USA. *Brit. J. psychiat. soc. Work* **3**, i, 4–12.

HARRINGTON, M. (1961). The integration of child therapy and casework. *J. Child Psychol. Psychiat.* **2**, ii, 113–20.

HOME OFFICE: DEPARTMENTAL COMMITTEE ON CHILDREN AND YOUNG PERSONS (1960). *Report.* Cmd. 1911 (Ingleby Report). London: HMSO.

HOME OFFICE: DEPARTMENTAL COMMITTEE ON THE PROBATION SERVICE (1962). *Report.* Cmd. 1650 (Morison Report). London: HMSO.

HUNT, A. (1962). *Enforcement in probation casework.* (Paper given at Generic Conference, London, 1962.)

IRVINE, E. E. (1959). Editorial comment. *Brit. J. psychiat. soc. Work* **5**, i, 2.

—— (1962). *What is advanced casework?* Barnett House Papers.

—— (1964). Mental health education in the community. *Brit. J. psychiat. soc. Work* **7**, iii, 136–41.

JEFFREYS, M. (1965). *An anatomy of social welfare services.* London: Michael Joseph.

JONES, K. & HAMMOND, P. (1960). The boundaries of training. *Brit. J. psychiat. soc. Work* **5**, iv, 172–7.

LEWIS, K. M. (1950). The role of the P.S.W. In report of the proceedings of the 108th Annual Meeting of the B.M.A., Section of Psychiatry. *Brit. med. J.* **ii**, 292.

MACINTOSH, J. M. (1951) *Social workers in the mental health services.* Cmd. 8260. London: HMSO.

MACKENZIE, M. (1963). Changing concepts in the field of child health. *Public Health.*

MENZIES, I. E. P. (1961). *The functioning of social systems as a defence against anxiety.* Tavistock Pamphlets no. 3. London: Tavistock Publications.

MINISTRY OF HEALTH (1959). Report of the working party on *Social workers in the local authority health and welfare services.* (Younghusband Report). London: HMSO.

MOFFATT, C. (1955). Communication. *Brit. J. psychiat. soc. Work* **3**, ii, 32–3.

RAFFERTY, F. T. (1960). Symptoms and process in the multidisciplined community. *Amer. J. Orthopsychiat.* **34**, iii, 569–75.

RICE, A. K. (1965). *Learning for leadership.* London: Tavistock Publications.

ROGERS, E. & DIXON, J. (1960). *Portrait of social work.* London: Oxford University Press.

SCOTTISH HOME AND HEALTH DEPARTMENT (1966). *Social work and the community: proposals for re-organizing local authority service in Scotland.* Cmd. 3065. London: HMSO.

SCOTTISH HOME AND HEALTH DEPARTMENT AND SCOTTISH EDUCATION DEPARTMENT (1964). *Report of the Committee on Children and Young Persons* (Scotland). Cmd. 2306. London: HMSO.

SIMON, H. A. (1965). *Administrative behaviour*, 2nd edn. London: Collier-Macmillan.

SOFER, C. (1961). *The organization from within.* London: Tavistock Publications.

THOMAS, E. L. (1950). The role of the psychiatric social worker. *Brit. J. psychiat. soc. Work* **1**, iv, 22–4.

TIMMS, N. (1964). *A history of psychiatric social work in Great Britain.* London: Routledge & Kegan Paul.

WOODWARD, J. (1961). Research and after. *Brit. J. psychiat. soc. Work* **6**, ii, 68–73.

7 The Changing Role of the Clinical Psychologist

HERBERT PHILLIPSON

Elsewhere in this volume, Dr Sutherland points to some changes that are necessary in the role of the psychiatrist to meet the wide range of tasks that the newer concepts and practice of community mental health present. He also demonstrates that boundaries between the skills and responsibilities of psychiatrists and those of non-medical colleagues need re-examination. And he foreshadows that any redefinition of roles and responsibilities will draw more from task experience than from history and tradition, important as these are.

I shall develop a similar view in discussing the changing role of the clinical psychologist. I shall give most attention to the role of the psychologist as it is, and as it may develop in relation to the growth of knowledge and skills deriving from and relating to psychotherapeutic work.

THE TEAM APPROACH

I shall build my discussion on the assumption that the wide range of mental health tasks requires a team approach; firstly, because of the complexity and the interrelatedness of the fields of knowledge they draw upon, and, secondly, because of their increasingly evident social content. If this is so, then the development of a rationale that can guide the structure and practice of the team in relation to its tasks is a prerequisite for the clarification of the roles and distinctive contributions of the several complementary disciplines within it. Stated in another way, the optimal development of these roles and contributions, upon which the health and effectiveness of the team depends, is itself closely bound up with the theory and practice of the team as a social-professional unit. To develop this theme I shall first refer, briefly, to the history and task of the mental health team.

The team approach had its origin in the child-guidance movement in the years between the two world wars. Its objectives
were to examine and help the whole person in relation to his
social and physical environment. In these early years the contributions of the members of the team to diagnosis and treatment
were sometimes well co-ordinated, but in general they remained
piecemeal. By the mid-1930s the beginnings of a more integrated
team approach were being sought under the influence of child
psychoanalysis, infant and child observation (e.g., by Susan Isaacs
and Piaget), and early studies in cultural anthropology. The
experience of the war years, with its breakdown of family and
social units, sharpened the recognition that the individual becomes a person, and maintains and extends his personality,
through his relations with others. This sharper awareness provided the basis for a shared body of knowledge, and a closer
fitting together of skills, through which this more integrated team
approach was developed in the post-war years.

In the adult area of work, the experience of a multidisciplinary
team approach developed within the war years in dealing with
'crisis' problems, largely in the Services. These included selection
of personnel for new roles, individual and unit morale, rehabilitation of battle casualties, the study of national character, and the
resettlement of prisoners of war. In Britain and in America, the
main emphasis in much of this work was upon the social influences that contribute to mental health and effective behaviour,
or to breakdown or maladaptive behaviour.

This emphasis on the psychodynamics of social systems was
shared within the wide range of disciplines contributing to the
work; psychiatry, psychoanalysis, educational and clinical psyco-
logy, cultural anthropology, and sociology. Out of this experience
came the development of group psychotherapy and methods of
community resettlement. Considerable impetus was given to the
development of projective and sociometric methods of studying
interpersonal relations. The value of some of the more structured
and so-called objective methods of personality assessment was
challenged, particularly when they were used without taking into
account the interpersonal and social factors affecting the data they
provided.

The experience of the war years sensitized many members of
the different disciplines to the social and community aspects of

mental health problems that could be foreshadowed as a result of the rapid technological and social changes during and after the war years. These problems, and the development of mental health services to meet the challenge they presented, were the main concern of the International Congress on Mental Health in 1948 (Flugel, 1948).

The social effects and concomitants of rapid technological advances are well known to us all. They include, for example, the changes of roles and relationships within the family; the break-down of many of the established networks connecting nuclear and extended family, family and field of work, work and com-munity, school and family, school and work; the isolation and lack of interpersonal expression in much of work and leisure activities; the breakdown of value systems and beliefs which formerly regulated interpersonal and group relations; the limita-tions of the social means by which responsibility may be taken and exercised in many key areas of life.

These, and related changes, bring about or increase mental illness in the individual and in the social unit. Work with family dyads, larger family units, and other social groups shows how fully the range and quality of interaction is subject to mutually maintained regulation within the social unit. Thus for example, in family mental health work the concern is not so much with the problem of husband, wife, or child in itself, but rather with the family as a whole and its own idiom of interexperience and interaction. The responsibilities for change, and indeed the mobilization of capacities for change, rest with the social unit, in its wholeness, as well as with its individual members. This concept of social functioning has its application in a large proportion of situations in all areas of mental health work, in treatment, prevention or positive mental health activities.

It follows, therefore, that professional work that includes a concern for the interpersonal and social influences in mental health, either as a basis for psychotherapeutic work with indivi-duals, family units, or social groups, or as a factor influencing the course of other forms of treatment, includes two requirements of the mental health team and of all its members. These concern

1 the principles governing professional relationship with indi-viduals and groups; this might be called the professional ethic.

2 the professional interpersonal and social skills necessary to serve this ethic.

1. *The Professional Ethic*

The aim is to optimize the participation of the subject in the mental health activity, and to optimize also his responsibility for decisions taken in, or in respect of, that activity. The mental health team is conceived of as a social unit, capable of conducting professional transactions with social units in the community around such explicit and implicit problems as emerge within the processes of social change. That its professional relationships are seen as transactions implies a reciprocity in the relationships between mental health workers and patients, in which responsibilities and decisions are as far as possible shared. It means that what is offered of help and understanding, within the safeguards of a professional relationship, provide the conditions under which the client may begin to communicate the content of social dilemmas, while in turn these communications provide the data and understanding through which the worker may more fully realize his professional role.

Stated more generally, changes, whether they affect the close interpersonal relations of nuclear family units, the group relations (small or large) in work or education, or the seeking for and adoption of new value systems, are, in predominant measure, the responsibility of the social units concerned. This is a desirable ethic from the viewpoint of society; it is perhaps the only proper and acceptable one. From the professional viewpoint it is not only desirable in principle, but also an essential component of mental health practice.

In practice, the application of this principle ensures the active participation of the subject in the process of exploration and change. Such participation, where the subject feels he has a stake in the outcome, is the surest guarantee of effort on his part, as it is of the acceptance of change, where this can be brought about. Any alternative approach that tends to rely on precept or advice, however well informed, is likely to meet with resistance, or may indeed intensify resistance by confirming in the subject his own feelings of helplessness and resentment at his incapacity to make changes through his own efforts.

The ethic, therefore, involves meeting needs as they appear, and approaching them at the time, and in the form, that engages the active participation of the subject. This approach, if successful, will mean that the range and depth of problems for which help is sought will extend.

It is within this ethic that the research and professional needs of the mental health team can be seen to be complementary. For example:

(a) It is only within a therapeutic transaction that access can be gained to the conflict-dominated areas of interpersonal and social interaction.

(b) To conduct research under these conditions means that the data obtained are close to the processes under investigation. This makes it more likely that the outcome of research will find ready application.

(c) Research effort of this kind keeps the mental health team and its members closely in touch with the full complexity of individual behaviour and social interaction, so that limited and facile investigations that do not do justice to the nature and complexity of the problems are rejected. The research worker will become aware that to impose a methodology upon his data rather than seek for one that fits them, may be not unlike the strivings of his patients to make do with a rationalization as a way of avoiding more painful issues.

2. *The Shared Component of Knowledge and Skills necessary for Mental Health Team Practice*

The context of social change within which mental health problems emerge, the nature of the tasks, the requirements of the professional ethic in relation to them and their method of solution, point to one component of knowledge and skills that is necessary for the practice of the mental health team. This should provide, within the team, a capacity to make direct professional contact with the processes of human interaction as they present themselves for help.

Without this training in the psychodynamics of human relations, the mental health worker too easily becomes a confused part of the problem he is trying to understand. Only on the basis of an awareness of the part he is given, or is taking, within the process he is treating, and a sensitivity to what this means, can he maintain and extend his professional or his scientific role.

This component of knowledge and skill should be shared by all members of the mental health team. Some will have more of it than others, because of their special interest and training. All will have sufficient of it to share in the overall responsibility of the team, which lies in its therapeutic commitment. Diagnosis or research, or teaching and supervision, or the support of caretaker services will be seen as social transactions in which problems are brought and help expected, indeed required, as a necessary part of these procedures.

Emphasis is given to this shared component of knowledge and skill because it is as necessary for a truly integrated team approach as it is for clinical work of the kind it seeks to do. Not only does such a common component of understanding and skill give each member of the team a part in its overall purpose, its therapeutic commitment, but it also provides the means for fuller and freer co-operation in the range of team activities. It offers also the possibilities of sharing and exchanging roles and responsibilities. These latter possibilities clearly have technical usefulness in work with family and other social units. In addition the experience of this common training provides a shared vehicle of communication, closely bound to the practical problems the team is concerned with. This invites and facilitates discussion of the data in terms of other theoretical constructs, which the different specialities in the team will contribute in their practice.

To emphasize the importance of this shared component of training for the mental health team takes nothing from the importance of the considerable range of knowledge and skills that are now a part of mental health practice. The intention is, rather, to emphasize the conditions within which the various disciplines that make up a team can optimize their contributions. It is argued that this common knowledge and skill provides one necessary condition for ensuring a fuller integration of the many approaches and areas of specialized knowledge used in mental health work, and for resolving some of the seeming conflicts that at present exist between them.

This appraisal of the mental health team is clearly particularly appropriate to the special centres that provide resources of consulting services, supported by research and teaching facilities, for a wide range of mental health activities and professions. Such centres give a setting in which the development of theory and practice can be tested out in a wide context. They also offer training resources wherein professional skills and patterns of co-operation between the disciplines can be experienced. This experience will inevitably influence the pattern of work in smaller mental health units.

THE DISTINCTIVE ROLE OF THE CLINICAL PSYCHOLOGIST

Within the context of such an appraisal of the task of the mental health team, it is possible to examine the distinctive contribution of the clinical psychologist and point to some possible directions for its development. His distinctive contribution will come from his graduate and postgraduate training in the knowledge and methods of general psychology and related sciences, built into a practical experience in a mental health service setting. Within this practical training his basic knowledge and skills are extended, often transformed, through experience of their application in dealing directly with human problems in a professional–scientific role.

It will be recognized that the heritage and tradition of general psychology that is one basic core of the clinical psychologist's training, is not static in its attitudes, content of knowledge, and experimental skills. Indeed the application of the content and methods of general psychology to problems of the individual, and of family and social groups in clinical practice, provides one important source of change and enrichment of the theory and practice of the wider discipline.

The scientific attitudes and skills that the psychologist derives from his undergraduate and postgraduate training in academic settings provide a basis for a distinctive contribution within the scientific component of the mental health team's work. How this potentiality can be realized through the application of these attitudes and skills in postgraduate clinical training depends on a clarification of the role and contributions of the psychologist in the mental health team. This clarification depends, in turn, on the resolution of two major dilemmas that confront the profession at the present time. Firstly, the seeming contradiction between his roles of scientist and clinician, and, secondly, the limitations and uncertainties within his role relationships with medical and other colleagues. The point of view developed so far in this paper leads to the possibility that these dilemmas are capable of resolution, and the role of the psychologist thereby capable of clarification, within the theory and practice of mental health team work, *which includes* within its framework the interpersonal and social influences on behaviour, and consequently includes, as a skill shared by all disciplines in the team, the ability to deal directly with human interaction. This point of view will now be applied in the examination of some important aspects of the psychologist's role and contribution in three related areas of mental health team activities: diagnosis, treatment, and research.

Diagnostic Work, Research, and Therapy

Potentially, diagnostic work offers opportunities that closely match the psychologist's scientific attitudes and training. Potentially also it brings him close to the basic objective in mental health activities, which is treatment in its broadest sense, including the preventive and positive aspects. In addition diagnostic work, closely related to treatment, offers the richest and most direct opportunities for making and checking hypotheses about the nature and operation of those structures and processes that make up human behaviour. That these potentialities are too seldom and too little realized by the psychologist is a responsibility he shares in large measure with other members of the mental health team. The realization of these potentialities requires an overlap of diagnostic, therapeutic, and research functions so that their inter-relatedness can be worked out in practice as well as in theory. The extent to which this can be achieved in the work of the psychologist will regulate the development of his distinctive contribution to the scientific aspects of this part of the team's work.

While the clinical psychologist has contributed much in the past to mental health work through his development and use of standardized test methods as aids in diagnosis, his role in this area of work has, by itself, become increasingly unsatisfying to him.

The psychologist and his colleagues have become increasingly aware of the limitations of standardized tests and procedures by themselves. Their greatest value has been seen in settings where there is close collaboration within the mental health team and where, at the same time, more subjective judgements by the psychologist himself and often by his colleagues add context and meaning to the more objective and indirect data from test procedures. But even where this is so, the scientific aspect of the psychologist's role is still challenged by his inability to understand, and find methods of controlling, the interpersonal and related situational influences on the reliability of the test data obtained so that their productive usefulness may be increased.

Clearly the integration of a psychotherapeutic approach within a diagnostic procedure in which psychological tests are used offers a way of examining this dilemma. The possible reciprocal value to the psychologist, in his dual role of scientist and clinician, of a participant therapeutic relation in such interviews has been little explored. For example, the considerable amount of work on the effect of the patient–psychologist relationship on test performances has not been exploited to help the patient understand why he behaves in the way he does in a particular relationship. By doing this the psychologist can explore more fully the nature of, and operation of, interpersonal variables that affect the reliability of test performances. For, indeed, the patient's problems are reflected in the idiosyncrasy of his performance and an essential part of the psychologist's task is to understand how and why such behaviour occurs.

To make progress in these directions the psychologist needs to adapt present concepts, and develop new ones, from psychodynamic theories of interpersonal experience and behaviour that can be used in diagnostic therapeutic explorations. In particular he needs the kind of experience that enables him to understand behaviour, including test performances, as communications in the interview relationship. He can then respond with therapeutic communications and see their effect upon perception, intellectual functioning, or learning in subsequent tests. Without this knowledge and skill psychodiagnostic work is subject to serious constraints. Any limit-testing methods used with cognitive, projective, or other tests will lack precision: resulting evidence about the patient's potential problems or positive resources, or his effectiveness in other motivational situations, will be too general and inferential; the patient's learning through the experience of the diagnostic procedure will be restricted.

Clearly where this skill in using an interpersonal reference is shared with other members of the mental health team, the formulation of questions to be explored by the psychologist in psychodiagnostic work, as well as the implications of the patient's experiences with him and with other units of the team, can be worked out more meaningfully. Communication within the team is improved. Differences of view and of data, obtained by different disciplines with their different methods and different relationship contexts, can be used constructively by the team to understand the patient's behaviour more fully, rather than as vehicles of interprofessional uncertainties and possible dissatisfactions or rivalries.

Psychotherapeutic experience leads to an important awareness that can be applied in psychodiagnostic work. This is the recognition that much of the primary stimulus values in any situation centres around the human relationships within it. The extent to which split off, unconscious perceptions, cognitions, and affects interfere with more appropriate behaviour in a situation depends upon the degree of fit between the 'internal' systems of interpersonal experience that the subject brings to it, in terms of unconscious wishes and expectations, anxieties, and defences, and the structure and meanings inherent in the 'external' world in which he is required to operate.

Such a formulation makes possible the extension of the use of psychodiagnostic techniques and the construction of new ones by the psychologist. It enables him to work out ways of exploring and controlling these interpersonal influences. The meaning of the stimulus structure and content of the test material used, and of the psychologist–patient relationship in the procedure, can be understood in terms of the dialectic between the issues of human relationship inherent in them and the patient's idiosyncratic ways of dealing with them. For example, where a particular test, or more often an item within it, matches, and thereby evokes, the activity of an unconscious system, the kind of inefficiency in thinking and expression shown by the patient will reflect the dissonant interpersonal relationship operating in the situation. Interpretation to the subject of this interference in his performance with reference to his superimposition of dissonant interpersonal issues on to the test item, and also upon his relationship with the psychologist, may often result in improved intellectual functioning.

Thus intellectual functioning is seen as the product of a total situation in which the psychologist–patient relationship, as the social context, is an important influence. Recent work in which two people, husband and wife, or parent and adolescent, were required to work out intelligence tests together, and together reach a solution, suggests an interesting extension of this way of looking at test performances (Harrower *et al.*, 1960). It was found that the scores obtained by these dyads were sometimes lower and at other times higher than those the members of the dyad obtained individually. A dyad's attainment in these terms could be related to the kind of interpersonal experience and interaction that typified their particular relationship to each other and, within an item analysis in the test sequence, to particular issues presented in the items that were difficult or impossible for the dyad to deal with. We all know from our clinical experience, and from seeing family, work, school, and other social groups in action, that very often the social unit fails to grasp the facts of a situation, or to deal meaningfully with them, in relation to the intellectual resources the group contains within it.

This holistic approach to the study of such dimensions of behaviour as perception, cognition, thinking, and learning, in which they are seen as expressions of the total personality or social unit in action, is often criticized as too time-consuming and too dependent on the clinician's skill and judgement. Yet, as Sanford (1966) argues, the criticism of those diagnostic or experimental studies that abstract part-functions is more serious, for, as he says, 'this strategy, because of its very nature, is bound to fall short of the truth. Not only does it avoid the big problems; it fails to achieve its own chosen goal, which is to establish general laws of behaviour. The main characteristic of such "laws" (as it does "establish") is their lack of generality. They break down as soon as a new variable is introduced into the picture. Since real life constantly presents new variables, or variables not taken into account in the laboratory experiment, such "laws" are most limited in their applicability.'

The development of psychodiagnostic work in this direction points to the need for psychologists to devise psychodiagnostic procedures wherein the stimulus values of setting, task content, and formal structure of response are more fully known in terms of the interpersonal processes they evoke. Such a development can take place only from a sharpening of psychodynamic theory by increasingly controlled experimental work in a diagnostic–therapeutic setting, in which the motivation of the subject and the professional position and skill of the psychologist can ensure a meaningful examination of the processes involved. Such a psycho-diagnostic procedure incorporates a research aim, the achieve-ment of which includes the understanding and control of inter-personal influences. This understanding, and the control of these influences, is achieved through making the psychodiagnostic procedure a therapeutic procedure as well, in which interpersonal relationships may be explored and attempts made to change them.

While such a procedure may be primarily concerned with answering diagnostic questions, the nature and extent of person-ality problems, and likely response to treatment, it is at the same time a miniature therapeutic procedure, an experimental test of the patient's capacities to make, maintain, and change his relations with others meaningfully. As such it offers important prognostic information about response to psychotherapy or more broadly to social readjustment. For the patient it offers a useful rehearsal and a motivating experience towards future treatment. In some cases it can constitute a sufficient therapeutic experience in its own right.

For the psychologist, psychodiagnostic work is the grass-roots of his knowledge of human behaviour. Out of it should come a distinctive contribution to the development of therapeutic work, as well as increased understanding and the development of skills necessary in research.

The psychologist's research attitudes, and his training in research design and methods, do not mean in themselves that he brings creativity in thinking or in research achievement to the team. Creativity is an individual or often a group achievement. It does mean, however, that he can contribute towards a research approach as an important component of the mental health team's work.

But in so far as the psychodiagnostic work of the psychologist is unsatisfying and unsatisfactory for him as a member of the mental health team, his research efforts to understand and predict behaviour, or response to treatment, will be limited in their usefulness. Research will tend to be narrowly focused on con-sequences, to the neglect of processes and causes.

A great deal of recent research work has been concerned with psychotherapy, the evaluation of its outcome and understanding of its processes. Only to the extent that the psychologist has a first-hand experience of its processes can he ask the right kind of questions himself, or work them out with his colleagues, e.g. by following the methods used by Malan (1963). Similarly he needs this experience so that he can work out ways of reconciling the clinical and therapeutic needs of the patient with the needs of research design and methodology. This kind of research often requires an active involvement in the process under investigation as therapist, co-therapist, or independent observer.

Thus the extension of the psychologist's contribution to the scientific component of the team's work in diagnosis and research is seen to depend on the closer linking of these activities with therapy. It is claimed that this might be achieved through the integration of an increasing measure of psychodynamic sensitivity and skill within the design and methods of these areas of work. Since interpersonal implications are an essential part of the patient's experience of such activities, and consequently an essential part of the concern of the diagnostician, research worker, or therapist, they constitute a common bond of concern and of understanding between the three activities, and also between the different disciplines that take part in them within the team. The three areas of work are too closely interrelated to remain the exclusive province of any one discipline within the team. They are indeed parts of a single process, although it is appropriate and usually necessary to place different emphases, in aim or in method, on one or other part of the process to bring it more sharply into focus.

Present formulations of the theory and practice of psychotherapy make it difficult to explore its processes by scientific methods. Potentially the distinctive contribution of the psychologist is in the extension of the scientific method in therapy. Clearly he must take part in therapy to make this contribution. He must take part also in order to be able to collaborate more fully with other members of the team who are engaged in therapeutic work. The understanding of the processes involved in therapeutic work, and the development of methods that are more scientifically controlled will come more surely from the interplay of a range of disciplines and knowledge in direct contact with the task, than from a position of sustained distance and detachment.

In discussing the development of the psychologist's distinctive contribution in diagnostic work it was argued that his lack of direct contact with therapy, and in particular the interpersonal experience inherent in it, faced him with a twofold frustration. As clinician, the psychologist's responsibilities are often out of keeping with his training – and indeed also with the intensity and breadth of demands made on the mental health services – and he is thus too often in a position of dependence rather than inter-dependence within the team. As scientist he is without the skill, and the access to the living processes of interpersonal behaviour wherein he might use it, to sharpen and adapt his own techniques of investigation.

Perhaps psychologists have not fully understood the nature of this twofold limitation in the development of their role. In settings where psychotherapy is largely used as a method of treatment, the psychologist has sought training and experience in this work, motivated both by the resulting increase in sensitivity to inter-personal meanings and influences upon diagnostic test responses, and also by the increase in personal responsibility and satisfaction the work offers him. In many instances the personal satisfactions and status of the role of psychotherapist have drawn the psycho-logist away from his psychodiagnostic role and from the scientific aims inherent in it. Potentially, however, these psychotherapeutic skills can be used by the psychologist to devise procedures that are at once psychodiagnostic and therapeutic. The structure of personality and its capacities for change can be systematically explored so that better focused, and more effectively therapeutic, work can be attempted and progressively evaluated within the procedure itself.

In settings where physical methods of treatment are more widely used, the psychologist has usually attempted to use and develop a scientific approach more closely related to his back-ground of academic training. He has become increasingly dis-satisfied, however, with the use of standardized tests because of their uncertain predictive value. Dissatisfied also with the limited responsibilities that the diagnostic role by itself offers, he has sought to develop methods of therapy that are more exclusively his own, derived from the theory and method of experimental psychology. So far 'behaviour therapy' has given little or no serious attention to interpersonal experience and behaviour within the patient–psychologist relationship during the diagnostic and therapeutic procedure. To this extent its rationale, its range of application, and its capability of evaluation are limited. It may well be that the importance of behaviour therapy is less in the usefulness of the methods it has so far devised, than in the opportunity it has created for psychologists to test out and develop experimental and diagnostic methods within a personal therapeutic relationship in which they bear a large measure of responsibility. The potential gain to the development of the role of the clinical psychologist is considerable; its realization requires the inclusion of clinical skills to understand and make use of the interpersonal influences of behaviour and to elicit more active and responsible participation from the patient.

In presenting this viewpoint of the distinctive contribution of the clinical psychologist and the development of it, the emphasis has been on the need for knowledge and skill, shared with other members of the mental health team, in using interpersonal experience, including its unconscious components, as an essential part of diagnostic, research, or therapeutic procedures. Such a view does not mean that all psychologists – or other members of the team – should have similar specialist interests, biases, or skills in other areas. Indeed diversity of special knowledge and skill is of considerable importance for the development of the scientific component of the mental health team's work. The increasingly manifest overlap between the biological and social sciences requires as much communication between them as possible.

Equally these views do not lead to any assumption that psychologists will all attempt, or achieve, a balanced participation in the diagnostic, research, and therapeutic aspects of mental health work. Personal preference and skill will guide them to give thought and practice to different areas of work. The demands of a developing service will also require varying degrees of overlap of role, or exchange of role. Such overlap, and sharing of roles and their responsibilities, need not prevent the development of the distinctive contributions of the different disciplines in the team; it can enhance their potentialities.

THE FAMILY AND COMMUNITY MENTAL HEALTH WORK

So far the role of the psychologist and its possible direction of development in relation to the heritage of psychotherapy and its extension into community mental health work has been discussed in general terms, putting most emphasis on the conditions under which his role may be more fully clarified and developed.

Brief attention to two or three areas of clinical activity will illustrate the point of view taken; it will also give some pointers to the ways in which the psychologist's work may grow in response to the challenges and opportunities that the newer social and community aspects of mental health work provide.

As a result largely of their concern with the capacities and abilities of the individual and the difficulties that arise in their development and use, psychologists have a special interest in problems that relate to adaptation in school and at work. Psychologists are now developing their more traditional approaches in remedial work for children with learning difficulties, and in guidance work for adolescents with vocational problems, in the direction of more overt psychotherapeutic techniques. The methods they are using incorporate the interpersonal theories and skills derived from psychotherapy, while making use also of techniques that come from psychodiagnostic experience, including the use of tests, that are particularly relevant to the understanding of difficulties in studies or in work (e.g. Boreham, 1967). Both kinds of problem often result from a failure to realize abilities and skills through the normal processes of self-expression and reality-testing in relations with others in past experience in home and school. Standardized tests or other test-type techniques, some designed for the particular difficulties of the patient, are used to provide opportunities for reality-testing in the context of a psychotherapeutic relationship, with the aim of initiating a process of learning not previously attained, or of enabling the patient to test out in an 'off-centre' situation, or even in fantasy, ways of overcoming difficulties that are not available to him, perhaps because of specific but inaccessible anxieties. For example, with a bright but retarded child or adolescent who has never given any evidence to himself or to others of his latent abilities, it is important that this evidence is given in his interviews with the psychologist. Sometimes this can be achieved through a combination of interpretative work, and the careful choice of a test in which his particular anxieties are less pressing. Sometimes a supportive, carefully graded limit-testing procedure will enable the patient to come closer to his potential level of achievement than he had previously been able to do. Such an experience in his interview not only increases the patient's motivation to work at his difficulties with the psychologist; it also constitutes a reorientation in his view of himself and of others. For the first time he knows from actual experience what his abilities are. Indeed, he can only know that his abilities really exist if he has the experience of actually using them in the context of a relationship in which it is apparent not only that he knows what he has done, but also that the other person knows and that both understand and accept this new awareness and some of its consequences.

Similarly – indeed, the situation might arise with the same patient – he may be invited, gradually and progressively, to test out in a fantasy situation presented in a projective technique, e.g. a picture, the feasibility of dealing with a relationship that arouses great anxiety for him, such as challenging an authority, i.e. putting him own powers up against those in authority.

These methods clearly overlap those used in experimental psychology.

The development of this kind of work by the psychologist meets a need that is increasingly important to the individual, the family, the school, and the community, as pressures from social change give more emphasis to these problems. In addition it opens up more fully an area of psychotherapeutic work that focuses upon key maturational issues. In the particular techniques it uses it adds something to the general body of psychotherapeutic skills.

But the psychologist will also be aware of the social context in which these kinds of learning and broader maturational problems have developed and are manifesting themselves. He will seek to understand the problems, or particular aspects of them, as part of the interexperience and interaction patterns of the family, and try, either by himself, or with other members of the team, to work with the family. Sometimes it will be recognized that work with the family is the most suitable and economical approach, as when it is directed towards loosening some areas of communication and experience that are preventing growth and limiting satisfactions in the family unit as a whole. For example: an adolescent girl found that halfway through her 'A' level course she could no longer cope with her key subject, English, because she could not face any task that required a critical or analytic appraisal of the works she was studying. Her inability to criticize, to put her view against that of others, and her anxiety about hurting or spoiling good things, were evident too in her attitudes to other interests, and their effects could be seen in test performances. In an interview with the patient and her parents, these difficulties could be seen and discussed as part of their interaction with each other during the interview. Their avoidance of any direct confrontation with each other that might be critical or hurtful had been intensified through their experience with an older child who was very severely handicapped. For the first time their feelings about this experience could be shared.

Just as the child's problems in maturation, or more specific learning difficulties, may arise from or be reinforced by experience within the family, so they may develop or be intensified within the social and work setting of the school. Increasingly psychologists are developing a role in providing consulting services to schools whereby the staff may be helped to understand more fully how these behaviour or learning difficulties arise, and to find solutions, appropriate to their own responsibilities and skills, for dealing with them.

Little interest has been shown by social science in school, college, or university as a phase of life whose content and social context can optimize the maturational possibilities of its pupils. This is a main theme in Sanford's *Self and Society* (*op. cit.*); how to create a socio-educational system in which there is the best balance between the content of, and means of acquiring, experience, knowledge, and skills, and the need of the individual to develop his own resources. While the responsibility for such experiments in education must rest with the educationists, the social scientist can play his part in consultations necessary to conceptualize the task and guide its operation. The clinical psychologist with his intimate knowledge of individual, family, and social aspects of growth and mental health could play an important part in facilitating such social studies and in evaluating their progress.

A range of opportunity similar to that available in the field of education is also open to the psychologist who is more concerned with the individual's readiness for and adjustment to work. Few psychologists will be able to acquire the knowledge and skills necessary to cover such a wide spectrum of possibilities on their own. With a team approach the psychologist's own special areas of experience can be supplemented by those of his colleagues in his own and other disciplines. Clearly, the part that the psychologist can play in community mental health, in its preventive and positive aspects, depends on a secure groundwork of experience in individual and family work, in which his ability to understand and deal professionally with interpersonal and group relations has been an essential part.

In discussing the rationale of the mental health team in relation to family and community work, two essential components of its practice have been suggested, first, the aim to optimize the responsible participation of the subject, individual, or group, and secondly, the skill to make use of the interpersonal implications of the situation and processes members of the team are working with. Clearly the application of these principles in the different social situations within the spectrum of family and community work challenges the patterns of thought and practice used in individual psychotherapy. In particular it requires adaptation or even radical changes in the way awareness of transference is used, and consequently it requires quite basic changes in the manner in which a professional role is exercised. Perhaps the greatest differences are those between the explicit therapeutic situations in family and group psychotherapy, and work with social groups, caretaker services, and institutions. In the latter use is made of psychodynamic sensitivities in a way that is more broadly educative (in the root meaning of the word), so that the group or institutional task becomes the main vehicle of learning and change.

But the extension of mental health work from the psychotherapy of the individual to that of family units, and thence to educative work with social groups and institutions, does represent a considerable technical achievement, which also offers prospects of important theoretical advances and openings for research.

In individual psychotherapy the emphasis is largely upon fantasy and projection, and the situation provides no directly observable control data on how the patient conducts his relationships outside the consulting room. The focus of attention is upon the content and structure of the patient's internalized systems of interpersonal experience. Reality testing, in the sense of bringing the patients' inner experience, or his experience with the therapist, into play with a person in his actual life-space – husband, wife, employer, co-worker – is not a built-in part of individual psychotherapy.

In family work, with parent and child or husband and wife,

the emphasis in psychotherapy is upon the idiosyncratic organization of the dyadic or larger family system. Thus the focus is much more on the interexperience and interaction of the patients in their actual life situations. What is more, samples of this interaction can be recorded or observed and attempts made to analyse the processes in terms of their form and content, distinct from, as well as in relation to, the inner systems of experience which are more readily available for study in individual therapy. This advance to family work then makes it possible to bring together within the psychologists' experience, and also in his theory-making and research, the systems of interpersonal experience that make up the internal world of the individual, and the systems of interpersonal experience as they operate in real-life situations. The range of possibilities are extended in work with other social groups. It is through these kinds of shifts in psychotherapeutic practice that the dilemmas that retard the progress of research in psychotherapy may be resolved.

These changes in the theoretical understanding and practices of the mental health team as it directs its attention towards family and community work, enables it to make use of concepts and methods from other social sciences and from relevant behavioural sciences like ethology. Equally, these sciences also gain from contact with the theory and practice of mental health work of this kind.

The development of the psychologist's distinctive contribution to community mental health work, requires the addition of more social science and ethology to his basic training. Although all members of the team will draw increasingly upon the social sciences for their training and work in community aspects of mental health, it is appropriate that the psychologist will do so more than others because their content and method, particularly in their scientific discipline, overlap much of his concern in general psychology.

In mental health work, concern with social units in their own right and as contexts needed by the individual for support, self-expression, and growth, opens the way to observational studies of social life in progress. It makes more relevant the findings and methods of ethology and it invites a fuller integration of phenomenological studies of behaviour with psychoanalytically orientated studies of the individual, the family, and society. The bringing together of these related but in many ways different psychodynamic approaches within the behavioural and social sciences, in work with a wider range of mental health tasks, offers promise of new and sharper formulations of theory and a closer application of theory to practice.

SUMMARY

Consideration has been given to some possible developments in the role and responsibilities of the clinical psychologist, and the conditions under which these developments might be facilitated, in relation to the heritage of psychotherapy and its extension into family and community mental health practice. It has been argued that the development of the psychologist's distinctive competences within the team is a product of a working relationship between knowledge and methods from the behavioural sciences and those clinical and professional competences in dealing with the interpersonal influences on behaviour that he can share with other members of the team.

It is maintained that the psychologist's distinctive contribution is towards the scientific component of mental health team work and some illustrations are given of how the extension of this scientific component is dependent upon shared experience within the team, in particular in its therapeutic tasks.

Much of the supportive, preventive, and positive mental health work with families, work and social groups, institutions and communities will be concerned with people and problems that need very much less direct medical responsibility than is necessary in hospitals and clinics offering the traditional services for acute or chronic mental illness. For this reason, and also because of the considerable increase of services mobilized in a comprehensive programme, by far the larger part of the social and community aspects of the work will be done by non-medical staff. The resulting more widely based sharing of responsibilities for the policy and planning of mental health work, and the greater responsibilities vested in individual disciplines for their own part in it, will provide an important condition for realizing their distinctive contributions. Thus within the mental health team encouragement of responsible participation, worked out by the team in relation to its tasks, will increase the effectiveness and satisfactions of its members and of the team as a whole.

I

REFERENCES

BOREHAM, J. L. (1967). The psychodynamic diagnosis and treatment of vocational problems. *Brit. J. soc. clin. Psychol.* **6**, 150–8.

FLUGEL, J. C. *et al.* (1948). Report of the International Preparatory Commission. In J. C. Flugel (ed.), *International congress on mental health*, Vol. 4: *Proceedings of the international conference on mental hygiene*, pp. 285–320. London: H. K. Lewis.

HARROWER, M. *et al.* (1960). *Creative variations in the projective techniques.* Springfield, Ill.: C. C. Thomas.

MALAN, D. H. (1963). *A study of brief psychotherapy.* London: Tavistock Publications; Philadelphia: Lippincott.

SANFORD, N. (1966). *Self and society.* New York: Atherton Press.

© Herbert Phillipson, 1971

8 The Congruent Society

GEOFFREY GORER

In this paper I want to advance the hypothesis that nearly all values are determined by the culture and institutions of society and to suggest connexions between certain types of values and certain types of psychological stress.

The other authors in this book who have discussed the good family, the good individual, education, and similar topics have – almost inevitably – taken for granted the values of the society in which they and I live and have commended attitudes and behaviour that are congruent with the values of contemporary Britain. This is of course completely justified if – but only if – we all remain conscious that we are discussing the values of a specified society inhabiting a specified territory during a stated period of time, and not human universals. Anthropological evidence suggests that there are very few generalizations that can be made about the values of all human beings living in all societies of all continents and at all ranges of technological complexity.

To take up again a subject on which Elizabeth Bott has touched, a concept such as 'the ordinary good family' has numerous cultural values implicit within it. For us a 'good family' consists of only one adult of each sex and their immature children; but for very many societies in the world – and, indeed, in our traditional slums and rural areas – this would be a very impoverished and deprived family.

In a great number of societies a good family would certainly include grandparents and in a sizeable number it would include either the father's brothers or the mother's sisters and their spouses and children. In such societies, and they include such great populations as traditional rural China and rural India, a good family is one in which there are as many adults as possible to share in the maintenance of the household and the care of young children; the bad family is one in which all this work falls on a single man and woman, either through the hazards of death and infertility or through quarrels that cannot be composed. In our 'good family' the strongest emotional bonds should be those between husband and wife and those between children and their biological parents; but in a considerable number of simpler societies the strongest adult emotional bonds should be between brother and sister; and young children should have closer bonds with their mother's brother than with their father, and sometimes with their father's sister, rather than with their mother.

These illustrations – and for the time being I do not want them to be considered as anything more – are examples of what has been called 'cultural relativism'. As social anthropologists use the term, 'culture' is a non-evaluative abstraction, and therefore almost entirely different from the evaluative use of the term as employed by Dr Winnicott. A short definition, which I think most cultural anthropologists would agree with, is that culture is 'the shared and learnt patterns of behaviour, values, and institutions that are peculiar to a given society at a given time'. Culture is an aspect of a society, not of a nation; sometimes the boundaries of a society and a political nation coincide; but in the contemporary world most political nations are composed of several societies, and in some instances a society is divided into two or more parts by political frontiers.

Culture is learned and so does not include the innate biological and psychological characteristics of *homo sapiens*. All non-defective human beings speak; and the potentiality of speech is an aspect of man's biological endowment; but the language that a human infant will learn is an aspect of the culture into which he is born; and each language structures the universe for its speakers in a fashion that is unique to the language. Hunger is part of man's biological endowment, and, on an abstract level, nutritionists can designate the components of a diet adequate to promote growth and maintain health; but appetite is an aspect of culture, for societies are capricious in the food they designate as suitable for human consumption, as most nutritious, or as most enjoyable; and the number of times people should be expected to feel hunger within the day is almost entirely defined by culture.

In an analogous fashion, there are institutions that are found in all human societies: but the form these institutions take in a given society at a given time is an aspect of the culture of that society. Owing to the long dependent phase of the human young, permanent and socially approved bonds between at least the mother and some male are found in all human societies, and in most societies the male is the presumed begetter of the child; but how the pair are selected and whether the bond is inclusive or exclusive depends on the culture. In some societies the choice of mate is extremely limited, dependent on the elaborations of kinship rules; in very many societies the choice is highly circumscribed; even in societies such as ours, which give verbal approval to completely free choice, to random mating, the majority of marriages occur within the same social and economic classes, between adherents to the same creed, and in the majority of cases between inhabitants of relatively restricted geographical areas. It is worth noting that our concept of the free choice of mate (apart from a very few consanguineous relatives) is one of the more uncommon variants of cultural rules regarding marriage.

All human children have to be educated so as to become efficient replacements for the parental generation; but the content of the education, and the people designated to impart this education, are determined by the culture of the society into which the children are born or in which they are reared. Education is a human universal; the designation of professionals, rather than specified kinsfolk, as imparters of education, would seem to be confined to societies that have elaborated their technology.

Only those societies whose marriage rules allow considerable theoretical freedom of choice can make 'falling in love' or 'object love' an expected experience in the lives of the great majority of their members and designate it a major value. In the greater number of human societies spouses are designated either by the cultural rules of kinship and marriage or by arrangements between the parents or parent-surrogates of the bridal pair. Sometimes attention is paid to the expressed preferences or aversions of those about to be betrothed; but the notion that those about to be married should be 'in love' or that 'being in love' should be the sole or main reason for entering into marriage is completely alien to the values of most societies so far studied by anthropologists.

In those numerous societies that make no allowance for 'falling in love' in their arrangements of marriage, people do still 'fall in love' on occasion; but this is nearly always seen as socially disruptive and usually as potentially tragic. Where it is not socially expected, 'falling in love' is statistically a rare phenomenon; in the Lepcha village in the Himalayas that I studied there were two couples 'in love' out of a population of 176; all four were, of course, married to other people; and their passionate involvements with one another caused more social disturbance than any other human activity during the period of my investigation or in the recent memories of my informants.

In our society, of course, we place an extremely high value on 'falling in love' and tend to deprecate a marriage based on any other motive. We act on the assumption that this is a potentiality of every 'well-adjusted' young adult; indeed the inability to 'fall in love' with a suitable member of the opposite sex is often seen as an indication of the need for psychotherapy. 'Falling in love' is still socially disruptive if one or both of the people concerned are married; but I think there would be a general consensus that 'falling in love' is the most ethical reason for divorce; overwhelming love should not be thwarted.

I have thought it worth while taking some time on this topic as it seems to me one of the most vivid illustrations of the fact that all our values are culturally determined; and secondly of the fact that cultural values are determined by social institutions. Only when we decided that marriages could be based on the free choice of the two people involved was it rational to establish 'falling in love' as one of our universal values. The evidence is slight – chiefly based on novels – but it does seem as though there were a two-generation gap in the nineteenth century between marriage based on love being considered appropriate for the middle classes and its extension to the other social classes within our society.

Not only are values dependent on the social institutions that support them and facilitate their attainment; values within any given society at a given time tend to be coherently and consistently related to one another; societies tend to be congruent; and one possible definition of a good society (from the point of view of its members) is one that does not embody mutually contradictory values.

The coherence of the values within a given society at a given time was first developed by the late Ruth Benedict in her famous book *Patterns of Culture*. This was originally published in 1934 and can be considered one of the truly seminal books of twentieth-century social anthropology. Today, the categories she employed seem rather crude: the Nietzschean 'Apollonian–Dionysian' dichotomy, and the gross psychiatric classifications of paranoid, cyclic, and the like; but her reanalysis of cultures in terms of the values that the different institutions of a society facilitate or frustrate, and of the characteristics that a culture rewards or reprobates represented a major advance in the interpretation of the data gathered by social anthropologists. This aspect of her thinking has been so widely accepted into social anthropology that the originality of her work at the time is now often overlooked.

The other aspect of her theory is still controversial, at least in this country. This was her insistence that a culture is learned by all the individuals who compose a society at a given time, and is not disembodied in such high-sounding concepts as the super-organic or the universal categories of Durkheim or Weber. Since she first adumbrated this concept very careful and detailed studies have been made of the actual treatment of children in different societies from birth onwards; in the first place by her colleague, Margaret Mead, who has studied and restudied identified people in Manus, in the Admiralty Islands, for thirty years, as well as babies in several other societies; by a number of her colleagues and collaborators, among whom I would include myself; and also by anthropologists who are qualified psychoanalysts, among whom George Devereux is outstanding.

Among academic anthropologists in this country it seems to be considered unsuitable, if not derogatory, for fieldworkers to pay systematic attention to the treatment of infants and young children; and of course this would distract the fieldworker from the meticulous recording and analysis of kinship systems and other institutions that are the principal preoccupations of contemporary British academic anthropologists. Outside this academic world some outstanding psychologically oriented work has been done, notably M. J. Field's study of rural Ghana, *Search for Security* (Field, 1960), and Morris Carstairs's investigation of high-caste Hindus in *The Twice-Born* (Carstairs, 1957).

On the basis of all these studies, some generalizations can be made. In every society – or, in complex societies, in each significant subdivision of the society – parents have clear but usually inarticulate ideals of the characters that they wish their infants to manifest when adult; and the customary treatment of infants from birth onwards is congruent with these ideals of adult character. Only exceptionally is this congruence verbalized; the treatment of infants is either traditional or 'scientific'; but when it is carefully explored the congruence can always be discovered. And although parents are seldom articulate about the reasons for treating their children as they do, in many societies they can state the untoward results that would eventuate were the child to be mishandled. Thus, in our own society, with the exception of the lower working class, there is articulate fear lest the child be 'spoiled' or too 'self-willed'; if you get parents to describe a 'spoiled' child you get a fairly articulate negative image of a character ideal.

Only in those societies in which parents are articulately conscious of the negative image of the 'spoiled' or naughty or antisocial child, and consistent in punishing or reprobating any manifestations of the traits that are feared, is it possible for the child to incorporate parental commands and prohibitions and so develop a strict conscience or superego. In many societies parents shrink from punishing their children themselves; in some, punishment is delegated to strangers, masked as supernaturals; in some, excessive praise for suitable behaviour is employed (rather than blame for unsuitable behaviour) as when a whole tribe of hunters will turn out to honour a little boy's first kill of a bird or tiny beast; and frequently the judgement of real or supposititious others is invoked in encouragement or discouragement, to evoke pride or shame. In yet other societies parents mete out reward and punishment in response to their own autonomous feelings, rather than in response to the child's behaviour: they will punish a child if it has momentarily annoyed them, not because it has broken a consistent rule. This type of parental behaviour, incidentally, seems to be characteristic of our traditional lower working classes and may in part account for their greater expressiveness and their customary inability to pursue long-term aims, which the majority stigmatizes as fecklessness.

Comparative material from a considerable number of cultures establishes fairly conclusively that the strict post-oedipal superego of classical psychoanalysis only develops when parents regulate their children's behaviour consistently. The existence of the larval superegos postulated by the followers of the late Melanie Klein cannot be determined by anthropological fieldworkers, for their manifestations seem to be restricted exclusively to the fantasies verbalized in psychoanalytic sessions; but the existence of the post-oedipal superego is constantly manifested in behaviour and in the verbalized standards by which the possessors of a strict superego judge themselves and their fellows.

This is a point of more than theoretical interest, for our preferred types of political and economic structures – democracy and large-scale commercial enterprises – depend implicitly on the citizenry involved having strict superegos, so that they will work reasonably industriously and honestly without constant supervision and checking, because they supervise and check themselves. When such strict superegos are rare or absent one is likely to find either large-scale corruption and peculation or very elaborate structures of supervision and control, both overt and covert.

The theoretical point, however, should not be overlooked, for it demonstrates the provincialism of even the most sophisticated psychological theory when all the observations are drawn from members of a single culture or of closely allied and mutually influencing cultures. Where Freud's theories depend on the physiological maturation of the growing human child and the psychological derivatives therefrom, he would seem to have been making statements of universal validity; but when they depend on parental behaviour and the values current in a given society at a given time – especially inarticulate values – then his theories are, inevitably, of only limited application. And even in the field of physical maturation he seems to have paid very little attention to skin sensitivity and none at all to the use or restraint of the striped muscles. Restriction of infantile motility by swaddling or cradle-boards is general in several cultures, but not in those from which most psychoanalysts' patients derive; nor are many Western children heavily overclothed, as is typical for Northern Chinese infants for about the first eighteen months of life. It is theoretically unlikely that these predominantly restrictive experiences would have no influence on subsequent psychological development.

It has been found convenient to distinguish cultures according to the psychological mechanisms on which they chiefly rely for controlling individual and social behaviour – societies that invoke the sense of sin, those that invoke shame or pride, and those that invoke guilt. In individual development these seem to represent three chronological stages. The sense of sin is probably pre-verbal, and is characterized by its all-or-none quality; either one is blissfully in the right, wrapped in the oceanic happiness of approval, or one is completely in the wrong, damned, detestable, and detested. It seems likely that all human infants pass through this stage; but the only society we know of where this sense of sin, of complete unworthiness, is invoked as the major mechanism of social control is the traditional peasant society of Great Russia. The sense of pride or shame depends upon the acquisition of speech; it is the voiced approval or disapproval of others that is sought or shunned; at a later stage of development such vocal approval or disapproval may be internalized, but this is by no means universal. Wherein this differs from the precursors of the superego and the sense of guilt is that parental approval or disapproval is not primarily invoked, but that of a larger group within which the parents may or may not be included. Among the Lepchas whom I studied, to give one example, the parents maintained an even attitude towards their children, and never punished them physically, or by withdrawal of love or food. When a child did something naughty, the reproach would be 'Nobody will love or help a child who does this or that'; 'Everybody likes children who . . .' Approval or disapproval was ascribed to the whole community, and in adult life it had to be voiced. The response to voiced disapproval was a suicide attempt, often theatrical but sometimes earnest; I heard of no suicide attempt that was not preceded by spoken reproaches.

Among the societies studied to date, some variant of the sense of pride or shame is much the most generally invoked mechanism of social and individual control. For us who have been brought up in a guilt culture, it is very difficult to empathize with members of a pride or shame culture. For us, in most cases, pride or shame are temporary pleasant or unpleasant feelings, not the principles that should guide our lives. Our admiration tends to be given to the individual who stands up for what he believes to be right, for the imperatives of his conscience, whatever the views of the majority or of the rest of society: these are the supreme examples of the autonomy Dr Winnicott listed as a sign of health. For the members of societies based on a sense of pride or shame it is inconceivable that such behaviour should be admirable.

The values of a society that invokes pride or shame as the

major mechanism of social control are likely to be congruent with one another and not mutually contradictory; and the goals by which public approval may be gained or public disapproval averted are likely to be within the reach of all or the great majority of the members of the appropriate age and sex. It not infrequently happens that the actions that will attract praise or avert blame are repugnant to our moral standards, particularly in those societies where a young man proves his valour by murder, by taking a head or a scalp, or where self-torture or cannibalism are enjoined. But unless we claim an absolute standard for our own system of ethics, I do not think such societies can properly be described as psychopathic or psychotic, for they do not appear to produce psychological conflict within their members. When the groups within which murder or cannibalism are forbidden become too small, as has happened in some New Guinea tribes, particularly those described by Dr and Mrs Berndt (1962), they can be considered evolutionarily maladaptive, for the societies were set on a course of mutual extermination.

Some of the societies that have set very high standards of courage or endurance, which their young men must manifest if they are to win praise and avoid shame, have devised alternative roles for men temperamentally or physically unable to attain these standards. The best documented of these alternative roles is the *berdache* found in a number of tribes of American Indians in the Great Plains. A youth who could not become a warrior had the alternative of transvestism, of dressing as a woman and acting as a social woman, even to the extent of getting married and going through pantomimes of childbirth. The accounts tell us that the *berdache* suffered from no disabilities or contumely; but the parents of boys were anxious lest their sons opt for this role; and the *berdache*'s 'husband' was considered to have a rather unduly easy time, since his 'wife' was likely to be stronger than biological women, and he did not have the trouble involved in looking after young children.

In contrast to the pride and shame cultures, which do not set up standards unattainable by the majority, guilt cultures inevitably set up absolute standards which nobody can attain. Parental imperatives are never modified: 'be truthful', 'be honest', 'be modest', 'be brave', and the like. Not infrequently parental imperatives are mutually contradictory, as when boys are enjoined to stand up for themselves and also not to be quarrelsome, or girls to be modest and also to be attractive.

Besides the inevitably unattainable and occasionally mutually contradictory parental imperatives incorporated by individuals, guilt cultures not infrequently develop institutions whose internal values and standards of behaviour are incongruous with the values and standards of behaviour demanded in other institutions. Thus, the United States, and several other democracies, have a dominant value of egalitarianism, that one man is as good as another, and disapprove of behaviour by which the richer or cleverer or more successful try to lay claim to a superior position; but in their armed services they demand strict subordination and superordination, a formal recognition and acceptance of inequality. Conversely, hierarchical aristocratic societies frequently subscribe to a religion that places emphasis on the unique and equal value of every soul. Or people may be enjoined to seek as much as they can for their wives and families, and not to seek more than their fellow-workers. When different values and different types of behaviour are enjoined on the same persons in different institutions of the same society, one can, I think, say that the society is incongruous; the built-in contradictions will inevitably produce psychological conflict for some of the society's members. Such incongruity is almost synonymous with the 'splitting' described by Professor Morris and commented on by Dr Sutherland.

This incongruity is much more likely to arise in societies with guilt cultures because of the absolute values of the internalized imperatives. All societies of any technological complexity develop institutions within which different types of behaviour and different attitudes are necessary; but no conflict need be involved if the behaviour which earns praise or averts blame is differently defined in differing social institutions; if males (for example) are enjoined to be good fighters or good husbands, not good men. The categorical imperatives of the strict conscience combined with social and technological elaboration would seem to imply an incongruous society for its members, with resulting individual strain and perplexity.

This is not the same thing as saying that societies with complex social institutions and an elaborate technology, civilizations in the common speech meaning of the word, inevitably produce neurosis. In *Civilization and Its Discontents* Freud (1930) drew all his illustrations from the civilizations of Western Europe with which he was familiar; indeed he wrote as if civilization was the prerogative of Judaeo-Christian societies, and perhaps of the societies of classical antiquity with which his reading had given him some familiarity – Egypt, Greece, Rome. He completely ignored the high civilizations of Asia, such as Iran, India, Japan, and China.

Although these civilizations have not been studied with the particularity one could wish – the most careful studies have all been of village communities, not of the towns – it seems as though none of them has developed the strict superego of Western civilizations; indeed even journalists recognize the overwhelming importance of avoiding shame on the part of the Japanese and Chinese by using the folk-psychology term of 'face'. In many ways this is a dangerous term, for it reduces the strongest motives of many Japanese and Chinese to something quaint and out-landish, which need not therefore be taken seriously. It does, however, imply a sort of recognition that the motives of these high civilizations – with a much longer continuity in the case of China than any European civilization – are not the same as those of the West. As far as I can tell, these societies are congruent for their members, and do not produce the same type of strain or perplexity as do societies with strict superegos and internalized imperatives.

Basically, I am advancing the hypothesis that societies, such as our own, which develop self-supervising superegos in most of their members, inevitably develop the incongruities – the split-tings, in Dr Sutherland's phrase – that may produce perplexities and neuroses in many of their members. I would suggest the aphorism that the price of autonomy is the susceptibility to neurosis; the price of intensity is free-floating aggression.

Here we come to the question of values, of individual values. Enough societies have now been studied where adolescence is undramatized, without family revolts or juvenile delinquency, so that, on an abstract level, we can write the prescription for a society without adolescent problems: this prescription is the lowering of all intensity – in personal relations, in religion, in art. Is the peace of mind of most of the population worth the price? I can answer for myself, but for nobody else.

Similarly, we can enormously lower the incidence of neurosis, of character problems, if we do not cultivate autonomy, if we do not ask individuals to stand up for what they believe to be right against all social pressures. Is this worth the price?

What I am convinced anthropological evidence shows is that you cannot have your cake and eat it, have an un-neurotic, gratified, un-anxious population and hope for high art, religious or erotic intensity, courageous autonomy. Some psychiatrists write and speak as if a psychological utopia was to be had with enough skilled psychological intervention – that you can keep the heights while eliminating the depths. To my understanding, this goes counter to the cross-cultural anthropological evidence. Certainly, individual misery can be alleviated; but I do not think the causes of misery can be removed from a society without changing it in many other ways – without, to my mind, impoverishing it. But this is a personal value judgement.

These observations may not have very direct relevance to the immediate preoccupations of psychiatrists, save when their clients come from exotic societies. Yet sometimes, perhaps, it may be useful to realize that the incongruities of our complex society, combined with our self-punishing superegos, inevitably produce some measure of conflict and perplexity in many of our citizens, but also the high art, the intellectual curiosity, the emotional intensity, the heroism that are the glories of our society in the minds of many.

REFERENCES

BENEDICT, R. (1935). *Patterns of culture*. London: Routledge and Kegan Paul.

BERNDT, R. M. (1962). *Excess and restraint*. Chicago: University of Chicago Press.

CARSTAIRS, G. M. (1957). *The twice-born: a study of a community of high-caste Hindus*. London: Hogarth Press.

FIELD, M. J. (1960). *Search for security*. London: Faber and Faber.

FREUD, S. (1930). *Civilization and its discontents*. London: Hogarth Press.